Preface

Assessment is the hallmark of the health professional. It is the ability to distinguish normal functioning of the human organism from the abnormal, and if the latter is discovered, to determine the gravity of the abnormality. It does not mean pinpointing the precise pathological process underlying the findings garnered at examination; the ultimate expertise for this function belongs uniquely to the physician. Assessment, however, belongs to all the healing professions. Sorting out the healthy from the unhealthy and grading the significance of any threat to the human person is an activity common to health professionals of whatever type; furthermore, it is the prime characteristic that sets the professional apart from the nonprofessional. Thus this book will be useful to any professional who wishes to attain a higher level of cardiovascular assessment skills, especially coronary care, intensive care, and emergency department nurses; nurse practitioners and clinical nurse specialists; nurse anesthetists; physician associates; and medical students.

A word must be said about the recent phenomenon in which we are witnessing appropriation by the nonmedical health professions of increased areas of assessment responsibility. Not very long ago, all but the most basic assessment tasks were performed only by physicians. In regard to the cardiovascular system, for example, the nursing profession limited itself to certain elementary inspection skills: palpating the peripheral pulses and commenting on rhythm and force, auscultating the apical pulse, and measuring the arterial blood pressure. Even these precious few skills were hard won, and there are still nurses among us who can recount the resistance they encountered from physicians when they first used the sphygmomanometer to measure blood pressure. Today, happily, the medical profession is more eager to share these skills with others, since benefits accrue to the physician—there are other hands now to bear the burden—and to the client as well. The benefits reaped by the client merit comment, for doubtless many who read this book will recognize the somewhat painful truth that we have shortchanged our clients with heart disease by insisting that only physicians perform higher-level assessment. Coronary care nurses, for example, after learning from this book that the earliest and sometimes the only sign of heart failure is a certain kind of cardiac sound, will be quick to realize the lifesaving potential

v

of being able to detect such a sound and will surely wish that they had had this knowledge to employ with previous clients. In our time, new health workers are bringing assessment skills to populations in rural areas and the inner cities previously little penetrated by the health care system. These new trends are to be welcomed, and it is my hope that this book will give impetus to this movement.

The structure of the book is based on *modules*, or units, that briefly treat a single, discrete topic. Included in the modules are brief text material, thematic illustrations, and self-assessment exercises. Modules 24 and 43 consist of review questions, and Module 44 presents a case illustration. The plan of the book is such that each module builds on the knowledge contained in previous modules. Therefore the reader who skips modules will find the text unintelligible. The reader who proceeds from the first module to the last, however, will be rewarded by acquiring, step by step, a knowledge of cardiovascular assessment sufficient to prepare the practitioner for "midlevel" responsibilities, that is, a level that would be expected of a nurse in an expanded role or of a physician's associate.

This book has been composed with the recognition that graduate professionals and students of the various professions will come to their study of cardiovascular assessment with differing health care knowledge bases. For example, critical care nurses may already possess a considerable number of assessment skills absorbed on the job and grafted onto a broad base of knowledge derived from the social and life sciences, and physician's associate students may be basing their study of cardiovascular assessment on their military training as hospital corpsmen and corpswomen. Since I have been both military corpsman and professional nurse, I have attempted to take both types of background into consideration. The only prior knowledge that the book assumes is a basic familiarity with the anatomy and physiology of the heart, fundamental medical terminology, and the ability to assess the vital signs, including the arterial blood pressure. Nevertheless, concepts that may be considered to border on the line between basic and more advanced are briefly explained to refresh the reader who has been previously exposed to them and to acquaint the reader who has not. (For instance, the physiological principle of Starling's law, which explains a number of signs in heart failure, is concisely reviewed at the appropriate point in the text.)

The principle that has guided me in preparing the content of the book has been the proverb, "When you hear hoofbeats, do not look for zebras." Thus emphasis has been placed on the entities one is likely to encounter in everyday practice. Uncommon diseases and complex explanations of phenomena whose origins are a matter of debate have been purposely omitted.

Grateful acknowledgment is made to the following staff members of William Beaumont Army Medical Center who volunteered their time to critically review the manuscript: to Lieutenant Colonel Joseph A. Paris, M.D., F.A.C.C., Chief of Cardiology Service, and Major Joanne Rollings, R.N., M.S.N., Critical Care Clinical Nurse Specialist, for their review of the manuscript in its entirety; and to

CARDIOVASCULAR ASSESSMENT

Guide for nurses and other health professionals

DONALD A. THOMPSON, R.N., M.S.N., F.N.C.

Major, Army Nurse Corps,
Ambulatory Care Clinical Nurse Specialist,
El Paso, Texas

with 126 *illustrations*

The C. V. Mosby Company

ST. LOUIS • TORONTO • LONDON   1981

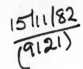

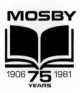

MOSBY

1906 **75** 1981
YEARS

A TRADITION OF PUBLISHING EXCELLENCE

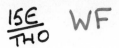

Opinions expressed in this book are entirely those of the author and do not necessarily represent Department of the Army policies.

The C. V. Mosby Company
11830 Westline Industrial Drive, St. Louis, Missouri 63141

Library of Congress Cataloging in Publication Data

Thompson, Donald A   1942-
    Cardiovascular assessment.

    Bibliography: p.
    1. Cardiovascular system—Diseases—Diagnosis.
2. Cardiovascular disease nursing.   I. Title.
[DNLM: 1. Cardiovascular diseases—Nursing—Problems.
WY 18 T469c]
RC670.T47   616.1'075'024613   80-26489
ISBN 0-8016-4954-4

C/D/D 9 8 7 6 5 4 3 2 1   01/D/040

Major Robert Anders, R.N., M.S.N., Psychiatric–Mental Health Clinical Nurse Specialist, Lieutenant Colonel Marilee Tolliefsen, R.N., M.S.N., Pediatric Clinical Nurse Specialist, and Captain Kathleen Walter, Pediatric Nurse Practitioner, for their review of those portions of the manuscript pertinent to their specialties.

Donald A. Thompson

Contents

CARDIOVASCULAR ASSESSMENT

Guide for nurses and other health professionals

MODULE 1

Taking the heart history: physical aspects

The physical aspects of the cardiovascular history must center on the four cardinal symptoms of heart disease: dyspnea, chest pain, palpitation, and syncope. Other symptoms that sometimes accompany heart disease are fatigue, headache, weakness, and loss of appetite, but they are all nonspecific and are seldom prominent in any given case of cardiac illness. Truly, then, the four cardinal heart symptoms form the very "heart" of the heart history.

DYSPNEA

Dyspnea is the general term for any difficulty with respiration, and it is the most common symptom of cardiac disease. There are four subtypes of dyspnea that are typical of heart disease: (1) shortness of breath, (2) cardiac cough, (3) paroxysmal nocturnal dyspnea, and (4) orthopnea.

Shortness of breath

Another term for shortness of breath is "breathlessness." This can be defined as the sensation of not being able to obtain satisfaction while drawing in a breath of fresh air. Defining shortness of breath in this way focuses attention on the *inspiratory* phase of respiration and distinguishes breathlessness of cardiac origin from other forms of dyspnea encountered in diseases of pulmonary origin (such as asthma and emphysema) in which the distress contains a large *expiratory* component. Shortness of breath is most often a manifestation of congestive heart failure (CHF). In CHF because the weakening heart cannot pump effectively, the blood dams back to the lungs, causing them to fill with fluid and thus preventing gas exchange. To summarize, inspiratory distress calls attention to heart disease, and expiratory distress calls attention to lung disease.

The following statements illustrate the way clients describe their experience of shortness of breath:

"I can't get the air in deep enough."

"The air sticks in my upper chest."

"My wind has been cut off."

1

"It's hard to get to the bottom of each breath."

"It feels like I'm smothering."

In evaluating shortness of breath, one must ask the client two necessary questions:

1. "What kinds of activities bring on the shortness of breath?"
2. "What makes it better?"

Frequently the person with congestive heart failure is not short of breath while at rest but becomes breathless when having to expend energy. This is known as **dyspnea on effort** (DOE) and is generally an early symptom of CHF. Another early form of shortness of breath in CHF is **positional dyspnea,** sometimes called trepopnea. In this form of respiratory distress the client breathes comfortably in most positions while lying down, but if the position is changed to lying on one certain side (usually the left), difficulty in breathing occurs until that position is abandoned.

As CHF advances, the person is able to do less and less without becoming breathless. The progression of the disease can be quickly assessed with the question, "What kinds of activities have you had to give up?" As the illness becomes more severe, the client begins to experience difficulty at rest. This situation is always serious and requires aggressive intervention.

Cardiac cough

In CHF the accumulation of fluid in the lungs in the early stages may be insufficient to cause frank shortness of breath but rather may manifest itself as a cough, which might be the only symptom. This type of cough is usually dry and tends to display one or more of the following features:

1. Occurs at night
2. Precipitated by lying down
3. Precipitated by exertion
4. Precipitated by turning to one side

Paroxysmal nocturnal dyspnea

Paroxysmal nocturnal dyspnea (PND) is a special variant of shortness of breath that is highly specific to CHF. In PND the client goes to sleep as usual without any difficulty. After an hour or two he or she awakens with a terrifying sensation of suffocation. The client then sits up on the side of the bed or goes to the window for some fresh air—maneuvers that utilize gravity to drain fluid from the lungs to the legs and feet. After a few minutes the distress subsides and the client goes back to sleep, usually for the remainder of the night. If PND is accompanied by wheezing, the condition is called **cardiac asthma.** This condition is very real, very important, and frequently confused with "true" asthma (reactive airways disease).

Orthopnea

When CHF becomes advanced, the person is unable to lie flat because of dyspnea, which is relieved when he or she is sitting up (the term "orthopnea" literally means breathing erect). When orthopnea begins, the client finds that pillows must be propped behind the back for sleeping and that the pillows increase in number as the disease progresses. Thus the question, "How many pillows do you sleep on?" provides a good way to assess the extent of the disease. Be aware, however, that some people sleep on more than one pillow for reasons of comfort alone, and thus it would be inappropriate to describe two-pillow orthopnea in someone who has slept on two pillows since childhood. In the severest form of orthopnea the client is compelled to sleep sitting upright in an armchair.

As can be seen from this discussion, the varying forms of dyspnea that occur in heart disease often begin with disturbances of sleep, and an excellent way to pick up early clues to the presence of heart disease is by asking the question, "How well do you sleep?" Avoid phrasing this question, "How do you sleep?" since this invites the reply, "I lie down and close my eyes"!

CHEST PAIN

Pain that originates from the heart is most often a result of **ischemia** of the cardiac muscle. In ischemic conditions of the heart the myocardium protests against the lack of oxygen to its tissues by causing chest pain. The two main ischemic conditions of the myocardium are (1) angina pectoris and (2) myocardial infarction (MI). Since both of these conditions have the same underlying mechanism, their pain is similar.

The typical presentation of ischemic heart disease is pain that is located directly beneath the sternum. The pain often has a **pressure** quality that the client may express by balling his or her fist and placing it against the center of the chest (Fig. 1-1). Words frequently used to describe it include squeezing, tight, heavy, expanding, strangling, pushing, gripping, and constricting. If the pressure quality is severe, the pain is said to be crushing. A common description is, "It felt like an elephant was sitting on my chest."

Another frequent characteristic of ischemic heart pain is **radiation** from the center of the chest to other areas, such as to the left or right arm or both, or up into the neck and either jaw. In a certain number of cases, however, ischemic pain will present atypically, that is, in other areas of the chest or even the upper abdomen or teeth. An old maxim states that ischemic heart pain may be found anywhere between the nose and the navel.

The pain of angina pectoris typically lasts less than five minutes and is precipitated by one of the "four Es":

1. Exercise
2. Excitement

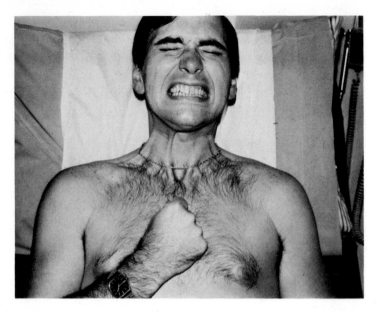

Fig. 1-1. Pain due to ischemia of the heart muscle frequently has a quality of pressure or constriction that the client is seen to express by clenching the fist and placing it over the center of the chest.

    3. Eating
    4. Exposure to cold

With rest, anginal pain tends to disappear. The pain of myocardial infarction, on the other hand, usually lasts longer than five minutes, often cannot be associated with any particular event, and persists even with rest.

    Another important type of chest pain is **pleuritic** pain. In this type of pain the membranes lining the lungs (pleurae) are inflamed. When the lungs are at rest in expiration, the pain is minimal or absent, but when the lungs are expanded in inspiration or upon coughing (or sometimes even during swallowing), the sensitive pleurae are stretched, which exaggerates the pain. This type of pain is usually noncardiac, but if heart disease inflames the sac that surrounds the heart (pericardium) at the area where the pleurae are contacted (pleuropericarditis), pain of cardiac origin may have a pleuritic component; that is, the pain will be worse when the client breathes in.

    A third common type of chest pain is **musculoskeletal** pain. Its hallmark is tenderness to palpation of the involved area of the chest wall. Another characteristic of this type of pain is that it is usually well localized, and the client can point to it with one finger or can trace the outer border of the pain with a finger.

    The fourth important type of chest pain is that due to **anxiety.** The location of this kind of pain is frequently in the left hemithorax or in the inframammary region, and the pain sometimes has a sharp quality, although chest pain arising from anxiety may assume almost any form and may even closely resemble that of myocardial infarction.

The sources of chest pain and common associated disorders are summarized below:

Sources of chest pain	Common associated disorders
Heart and pericardium	Ischemic heart pain Pericarditis
Lungs and pleurae	Pulmonary embolism Pneumonia Pleurisy Pneumothorax
Muscles and skeleton	Costochondritis Myositis Herpes zoster "Stitch"
Aorta and mediastinum	Aortic aneurysm (dissecting)
Upper gastrointestinal tract	Esophagitis Gastritis Hiatal hernia Cholecystitis
Anxiety	Polymorphous chest pain

Like all other kinds of pain, chest pain has five dimensions that must be ascertained while taking the history. These five dimensions can be recalled by the initials *PQRST,* as given by DeGowin and DeGowin (1976). The specific order is not necessarily followed, but the initials help the interviewer to avoid the omission of an aspect essential to assessment of the pain.

P = Provocative-palliative factors

Provocative factors are those which answer the questions, "What brought on the pain?" and, "Is there anything that makes it worse?" Palliative factors are those that relieve or remove the pain. Specific areas to assess in chest pain are the effects of (1) exertion, (2) rest, (3) breathing in or coughing, (4) position, (5) movement, (6) heat, (7) cold, (8) food, and (9) drugs such as nitroglycerin, analgesics, and antacids.

Q = Quality

Adjectives should be elicited from the client so that the nature and characteristics of the pain can be described. The following are five general qualities that (any) chest pain may have and some common adjectives associated with them:
   1. Pressure: squeezing, tight, heavy, expanding, strangling, pushing, gripping, constricting

2. Temperature: hot, burning, stinging, acid
3. Sharpness: stabbing, pricking, drilling, boring
4. Dullness: sore, pounding, gnawing, like gas, cramping
5. Tearing: ripping, pulling, splitting, bursting

Keep in mind that there may be some combination or overlapping of these qualities in any individual episode of chest pain and that the client may even use words that are contradictory to describe the pain.

R = Region

Describe the area of the chest where the pain is felt. Ask the client whether he or she can localize the pain with one finger. If the pain can definitely be localized with one finger, it is probably not ischemic pain, which is diffuse and localizes poorly. The client with ischemic pain is more likely to demonstrate the pain by using the closed fist, as already mentioned, by clutching the chest, or by using rubbing motions of the whole hand. The R for region should also bring to mind R for radiation.

S = Severity

Pain of any kind is difficult to grade. The most meaningful categories are "severe" and "less than severe." The latter category is sometimes expressed as "mild to moderate."

T = Temporal characteristics

The temporal characteristics include the pain's duration, its development over the course of time, and its periodicity (when it waxes and wanes).

There are two essential observations to be made about chest pain: (1) Non-cardiac chest pain may mimic cardiac chest pain. (2) Cardiac chest pain may mimic noncardiac chest pain. A corollary of the first observation is that no harm is ever done by considering a cardiac origin for a pain that turns out to be some other kind. The corollary of the second observation is called the Cardinal Principle of Chest Pain, which states: **All chest pain is myocardial infarction until proved otherwise.** This rule must be followed regardless of the region or quality of the pain. Although MI usually presents with ischemic pain, it can present in numerous atypical ways and can masquerade as various entities from heartburn to respiratory disease. Furthermore, each new episode of chest pain must be treated as though it were a new MI, even if the pain is identical to the previous episode, in which it had been ruled out.

PALPITATION

Palpitation is defined as an unpleasant awareness of the heartbeat when the subject is at rest or performing basal activities. The source of palpitations is premature beats and other rhythm disturbances. Perhaps the most common palpitation is simple overawareness of a normal sinus* tachycardia due to anxiety. Representative descriptions of palpitations are as follows:

"It felt like my heart jumped."

"My heart skipped [or dropped] a beat."

"A fish flopped over inside my chest."

"Suddenly my heart began to thump [or pound or flutter]."

It may be helpful to have the client tap out the rhythm with one finger on a tabletop to identify the pattern of the underlying arrhythmia.

Fortunately, palpitations are not often signs of serious heart disease, but health care providers need to inquire about two important considerations:

1. *Are they the result of* **life-style?** A frequent factor in the production of palpitations is stress. Cardiac stimulants such as caffeine and nicotine are often involved, as is the lack of proper rest. The classic example is the college student, cramming for final examinations, who gulps coffee and furiously puffs cigarettes while burning the midnight oil.

2. *Are they the result of* **drug toxicity?** Certain drugs, especially cardiac agents, if taken in excessive amounts, may precipitate arrhythmias that are experienced by the client as palpitations. This is especially true in the case of digitalis, since the range between its therapeutic effect and its toxic effect is rather narrow. Thus a complete drug history is essential in the complaint of palpitations. Incidentally, not all arrhythmias are symptomatic—some people are not even aware of lethal arrhythmias such as ventricular tachycardia.

SYNCOPE

Although the origin of most syncope is *not* the heart, a significant proportion of temporary loss of consciousness can be traced to heart disorders. If the heart does not perform its function as a pump adequately, the brain is not perfused with oxygen, and fainting results. Following is a discussion of four important types of cardiac syncope.

Effort syncope

Effort syncope refers to a transient loss of consciousness that occurs shortly after heavy activity is undertaken. The subject faints and, after several moments, arouses spontaneously. This syndrome is frequently caused by aortic or subaortic stenosis. In these two conditions, either the aortic valve or the area just below it is narrowed, and thus the amount of blood flowing past the aortic valve to the various parts of the body is reduced. As long as the client's brain and body have a low oxygen requirement, sufficient blood reaches the brain through the stenosed valve or subaortic channel to keep this organ adequately perfused. As soon as the client begins to exercise, however, the body's demand for oxygen outstrips

---

*"Sinus" in this case refers to the origin of the rhythm in the sinoatrial node (natural pacemaker).

the limited supply, the brain does not receive enough oxygen, and fainting occurs.

Stokes-Adams attack

A Stokes-Adams attack is a dramatic loss of consciousness caused by heart block or related rhythm disturbances. The client, usually elderly, faints suddenly and without warning, quickly assuming an ashen, deathlike appearance. There is no pulse, and the pupils may be dilated. Breathing may or may not continue. If the attack lasts longer than 15 seconds, convulsions may follow. If the attack does not spontaneously cease after this time, there is danger of total cardiorespiratory arrest and death. The attacks generally last for only a few seconds and are sometimes so brief they may be mistaken for petit mal seizures. When the heart reverts to normal sinus rhythm, the client regains consciousness rapidly, often accompanied by an intense flushing of the face.

Pacemaker syncope

Pacemaker syncope is caused by malfunction or failure of an artificial pacemaker. With more than a quarter of a million Americans having electronic pacemakers, and new implants being inserted at an estimated 30,000 per year, this form of cardiac syncope has become important. The mechanical status of the device must always be checked in someone with a "pacer" who faints, even if recovery is immediate.

Hypersensitive carotid sinus syncope

Hypersensitive carotid sinus syncope is usually found in elderly persons whose carotid arteries have become hardened by atherosclerosis. When pressure is applied on a carotid sinus body (located just below the angle of the jaw) of someone with this syndrome, an exaggerated vagal response occurs, manifested by a sharp drop in the arterial BP or even **cardiac arrest.** The client typically "passes out" when twisting the neck while shaving or when buttoning a tight collar. The heart generally "escapes" in a matter of seconds, but occasionally it fails to generate any escape rhythm, and death results. The risk of precipitating a fatal rhythm disturbance from an irritable sinus is sufficiently great that even when therapeutic carotid sinus massage is performed, it is never done on both sides at the same time on anyone. Cultivate the habit of examining the carotids **one at a time.** Furthermore, the danger of lethal carotid compression is increased in the client who takes **digitalis,** surely one of the most common medications taken by the elderly population.

EXERCISE *(see Appendix E for answers)*

1. The difficulty in dyspnea of cardiac origin usually occurs in the _____ phase of respiration.

2. PND accompanied by wheezing is termed _____.

3. PND is highly specific to _____.

4. List the two main ischemic conditions of the heart:

   a. _____

   b. _____

5. Ischemic heart pain often has a _____ quality to it.
6. List the "four Es" of angina.

   a. _____

   b. _____

   c. _____

   d. _____

7. Chest pain made worse by inspiration or coughing is termed _____.
8. List the five dimensions of pain.

   a. _____

   b. _____

   c. _____

   d. _____

   e. _____

9. All chest pain is _____ until proved otherwise.

10. Drug toxicity from _____ is an important cause of palpitations.

11. Effort syncope is frequently due to stenosis or narrowing of the _____ valve or outflow tract just below this valve.

12. A sudden, deathlike loss of consciousness associated with convulsions and flushing is called a _____ attack.

MODULE 2

Taking the heart history: psychosocial aspects

No assessment of a cardiac client can ever by complete if the psychosocial factors that play a role in the illness are not identified and evaluated.

SOCIAL FACTORS

To neglect the social context in which heart disease is found may help to perpetuate it. Examples are the client with rheumatic heart disease who has no transportation to go for monthly penicillin injections or the client with chronic CHF who cannot afford to buy low-sodium foods that may be beneficial in helping to cope with the condition. Does the overcrowded and unhygienic home environment of the client predispose to rheumatic fever? Does the client with valvular disease live in a milieu of drug traffic that renders him or her susceptible to possible bacterial endocarditis transmitted via contaminated needles?

The following questions are an integral part of every client's history:

"What is your income per month (year)?"

"Do you have any unusual expenses?"

"What kind of home do you live in? How many rooms? Does it have electricity and running water?"

"Do you have transportation?"

It may even be important in certain circumstances to inquire whether the client owns pets, since a recent study by Friedmann and associates (1979) has correlated survival after myocardial infarction (MI) with pet ownership.

The socioeconomic status of the client may have a bearing on how cardiac illness is perceived. For instance, it is common for persons at lower socioeconomic levels to view an MI as creating a permanent hole in the heart.

PSYCHOLOGICAL FACTORS

Certain psychological factors are particularly operative in heart disease. They include denial, depression, anxiety, stress, and personality.

Denial

Denial is a normal coping mechanism. We all use it, whenever we must do something risky (e.g., driving at night in the rain), by minimizing the bad consequences that may result and reassuring ourselves that all will turn out well. Denial indeed may help one recover from heart disease by "blocking out" an undue fear of it. This mechanism becomes pathological only when it is carried to the point where one denies that the illness itself has occurred or denies the feelings that are normally attached to the illness, such as fear, anger, and anxiety. An example of one who overuses denial (pathological denial) is the victim of an MI who tries to kill the pain with several shots of whiskey or, worse still, attempts a flight to health by trying to "jog it off."

Depression

Whenever people are informed that they have myocardial infarction, heart failure, or valve disease that will require open-heart surgery and lifelong anticoagulation with a drug also used as rat poison (warfarin), the inevitable result is depression. Depression follows the onset of heart disease as surely as pain follows a surgical incision. This depression often lifts by itself as adjustment to the illness is made, but if it is marked or long lasting, psychiatric intervention may be indicated. Although many instances of depression can be recognized by the sad facial expression and the "blue" tone of voice, some are not so obvious. The following are subtle indications that a depression may be occurring:
1. Change in appetite (usually decreased)
2. Change in sexual interest (usually decreased)
3. Change in weight (usually decreased)
4. Unusual brevity of speech
5. Early-morning awakening
6. Irritability
7. Indecisiveness

In some individuals with MI or other heart disease, depression does not take place while the client is in the hospital, but is "saved up" for shortly after the return home. This is termed **homecoming depression.**

Anxiety

Disease of the heart often engenders a diffuse anxiety that is out of proportion ot the actual severity of the threat to the client's health. This anxiety is commonly manifested by restlessness, muscle tension, and difficulty in thinking and concentration. Some anxious clients, however, present a calm exterior, but their anxiety expresses itself more subtly as multiple, vague physical complaints.

Few illnesses provoke more anxiety than heart disease; thus it is important to watch for the effects of anxiety on the history of any client in whom a heart problem is known or suspected. Anxiety may distort the history and mislead the practitioner about the nature of the problem. The two important effects of anxiety on the history are (1) embellishment and (2) omission. The "embellisher" relates

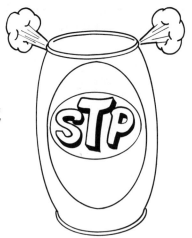

Fig. 2-1. Histories taken on clients with heart disease frequently indicate excessive amounts of STP (stress/tension/pressure).

such a wealth of detail about his subjective experiences that it may be difficult to sort out what is meaningful from what is insignificant. The "omitter" simply forgets to mention or represses important pieces of information.

Stress

Inquiries about stressors in the life of the heart disease client frequently yield numerous positive responses. The exact role of stress in producing cardiac illness has not yet been defined, but there is considerable evidence that chronic stress can produce physiological changes that may lead to heart disease. For example, income tax accountants in the period around April 15 have higher blood cholesterol levels, and rats who have to fight other rats for food develop higher rates of hypertension and coronary artery disease (Williams, 1979). Histories taken on people with heart conditions commonly indicate an excess of stress/tension/pressure (STP) in their lives (Fig. 2-1). Some studies have shown a high rate of life changes, such as death of a loved one, divorce, or change of job, in the period just before the onset of severe cardiac illness (Garrity and Marx, 1979). The military history of heart clients often turns up instances of combat and other extremely stressful assignments that may have played a contributing role. In any case, since it is an established fact that stress can retard recovery, every attempt to identify current stressors must be made so that they can be eliminated or reduced.

Personality

Considerable research is being done on the role of personality in heart disease. Friedman and Rosenman (1974) have described the coronary-prone personality, which they define in terms of the type A behavior pattern. To quote these authors, "It is a particular complex of personality traits, including excessive competitive drive, aggressiveness, impatience, and a harrying sense of time urgency." The type B personality has the converse behavior pattern—essentially the relaxed individual who does not display the type A characteristics. Cromwell and associates (1977), in a study of 229 victims of MI found that certain personality factors (high rate of information processing, perfectionism, bottling up of tension, denial of hostility, low mood for social affection, etc.) were more powerful predictors of a second MI than were clinical symptoms, blood tests, or the ECG. Although there are difficulties with any personality typology, the type A or B typology has gained wide recognition for its utility in describing a cluster of characteristics believed by many professionals to figure in the etiology of heart disease.

FAMILY DYNAMICS

Disturbed family relationships can aggravate the symptoms of cardiac illness. For example, hostile relations between the client with angina and the spouse or children may precipitate episodes of chest pain. The way in which the client's heart disease impacts on other members of the family also must be assessed. Family members sometimes overprotect one who has a heart condition, and if it so happens that the client has strong needs for dependency, he or she may limit activity below the level truly imposed by the disease. The decreased activity eventually causes the client's condition to deteriorate to such a degree that in the end, he or she becomes the very thing the family tried to prevent—an invalid.

A not infrequent occurrence after MI is the "sexual cripple" phenomenon, which can result if sexual counseling is neglected. In this phenomenon the couple remains sexually abstinent for an undue length of time (sometimes permanently) out of the erroneous belief that sexual stimulation in general and orgasm in particular are likely to provoke a second heart attack. The phenomenon has three manifestations:

1. Victim desires to resume, but spouse is afraid. Tactics used by the spouse to enforce the cripple role on the victim are evasion ("keeping busy") and keeping the victim at bay with warning statements such as, "You know the doctor said straining would be bad for your heart."

2. Victim is afraid, but spouse desires to resume. The lack of sexual activity on the part of the victim may stem from depression which is so common in the post MI client, as indicated previously. However, inactivity may also result from misinformation that sex after a heart attack is dangerous. It is to be emphasized that this situation, as well as the preceding manifestation, inevitably results in *stressful* relationships between the two partners.

3. Both victim and spouse are afraid. This manifestation is perhaps less stressful than the two foregoing situations, but it is certainly no less tragic.

EXERCISE *(see Appendix E for answers)*

1. Depression may manifest itself as _____ awakening.

2. Anxiety may express itself subtly as multiple, vague _____ complaints.

3. Inability to relax during leisure or wait patiently is a characteristic of the type _____ behavior pattern.

4. In assessing family dynamics in heart disease, one must look for any tendency of the family to _____ the client.

5. In taking the heart history, it is necessary to watch for the two major effects of anxiety on the history, which are _____ and _____.

MODULE 3

Some important physical signs in heart disease

Whenever hemoptysis, dependent edema, cyanosis, or clubbing is encountered during physical examination, the heart must be considered as a possible source. Although these signs sometimes have other causes besides the heart, they are of special interest because of the tendency to overlook their cardiac origin.

HEMOPTYSIS

Although most instances of hemoptysis have their origin in the respiratory system, there is one important cardiac cause: mitral stenosis (MS). In MS the left atrium has difficulty forcing blood through the stenosed (narrowed) mitral valve, which causes a rise in pressure inside the atrium. As the disease progresses and the valve opening becomes smaller, the increased pressure is transmitted through the pulmonary veins into the pulmonary vascular beds. Because of the high pressure in the pulmonary vessels in this condition, some of them rupture, causing the client to cough up blood.

DEPENDENT EDEMA

In dependent edema the fluid tends to accumulate in the lowest parts of the body because of the effect of gravity (in contrast to nondependent edema, which is not affected by changes in position). Dependent edema is a feature of right-sided CHF. When the right side of the heart fails, blood "dams back" through the systemic veins, causing fluid to waterlog the peripheral subcutaneous tissues. In an ambulatory client, gravity drains the edematous fluid to the feet, ankles, and pretibial areas. A good way to discover early dependent edema in such a client is by asking the question, "Have you had any trouble lately putting your shoes on?"

Edema is assessed by means of pitting, which is the ability to indent the skin when it is pressed with the fingertips. Normally the skin springs back immediately, and no indentation can be seen. The degree of pitting is traditionally rated on a four-grade scale:

    0 = absent
    +1 = Trace; disappears rapidly

+2 = Moderate; disappears in 10 to 15 seconds
+3 = Deep; disappears in 1 or 2 minutes
+4 = Very deep; may be seen after 5 minutes

In addition, the higher up the leg pitting can be found, the worse the condition.

In assessing the client at bed rest, avoid the pitfall of checking only the legs and concluding that there is no edema. The effect of gravity on edema in the bedfast person is to redistribute fluid from the lower extremities to the entire dorsal area; thus edema no longer shows so readily. To find dependent edema on the person who has been in bed, press over the sacrum, buttocks, and posterior thighs.

CYANOSIS

Cyanosis is of two types: peripheral and central.

Peripheral cyanosis

Peripheral cyanosis is characterized by a bluish discoloration appearing on the extremities, earlobes, tip of the nose, and lips, but *not* on the inside of the mouth. The most common cause of peripheral cyanosis is a **cold room.** Therefore, before concluding that abnormal cyanosis is present, ensure that the client is warm and comfortable.

Central cyanosis

Central cyanosis is generally the more serious type and is distinguished by blueness of the tongue and insides of the cheeks. The extremities may or may not be blue. Central cyanosis is associated with pulmonary disease that prevents blood from picking up oxygen in the lungs and with right-to-left intracardiac or intrapulmonary **shunts,** which short-circuit the flow of blood past the lungs. (A shunt is defined as a channel through which venous blood enters the arterial blood without being oxygenated in the lungs. For assessment features in congenital shunts, see Module 42: Cardiac Assessment in Children.)

CLUBBING

Clubbing is a rather mysterious phenomenon in which the tips of the fingers become enlarged and bulbous, usually in response to some underlying systemic disease. It is most often associated with pulmonary and cardiac illnesses. Of the latter, congenital cyanotic heart disease is most frequently associated. In advanced clubbing the fingers assume a drumstick appearance, but in the beginning stages they appear normal. There are two indicators of early clubbing: the floating nail and the profile sign.

Floating nail

In health the nail is firmly anchored in the nailbed, but as the process of clubbing gets underway, the tissues of the bed become soft and spongy. This

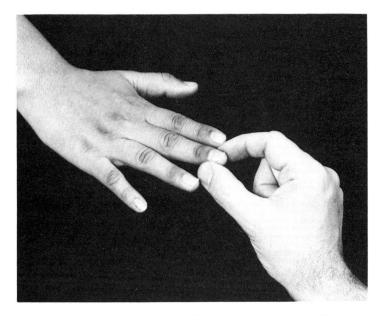

Fig. 3-1. Palpating the nailbed to detect floating nail.

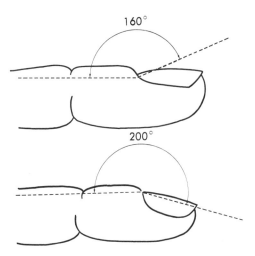

Fig. 3-2. Profile sign. Early clubbing sometimes evidenced by a nail-to-nailbed angle of more than 180°. Top view is normal and bottom view is abnormal.

condition, known as floating nail (Fig. 3-1), can be palpated in the tissues surrounding the nail. If the nail is pressed downward, it will spring back when the pressure is released.

Profile sign

When the finger is viewed from the side, take note of the angle of the nail to the base of the nail. This angle is normally about 160°. When clubbing begins, the distal edge of the nail begins to dip downward, so that this angle **increases.** Such an angle of more than 180° is generally considered abnormal (Fig. 3-2).

EXERCISE (*see Appendix E for answers*)

1. The one important cardiac cause of hemoptysis is _____.

2. Dependent edema is a feature of _____ CHF.

3. A pit remaining on the skin after more than 1 minute would be grade +_____ .

4. Merry Hart, a 5-year-old girl with congenital heart disease, is found to have a blue color on the mucosa of the inside of her cheeks. This condition is known as

   _____ cyanosis.

5. Merry should be evaluated for the presence of associated clubbing. The two indicators of early clubbing are _____ and

   _____ .

6. When Merry's fingers are examined, an abnormal angle between the nail and the base of the nail is found. It can be said that this angle must therefore be more than

   _____° .

MODULE 4

The four techniques of cardiovascular assessment

The four ancient techniques of physical examination are
1. Inspection
2. Palpation
3. Percussion
4. Auscultation

These four methods have stood the test of time and are used to this day on almost all the body systems. The one important exception is the cardiovascular system. In recent times the four steps for assessing the heart have been changed as follows (Fig. 4-1):
1. Inspection
2. Palpation
3. Auscultation
4. Contemplation

Note that percussion has been deleted from the list of modern-day techniques. It is useful only indirectly in the assessment of the heart. Two observations may be made about the techniques of assessment:

1. No technique must ever be omitted. To leave out a step is to risk missing a significant finding. For example, a gallop rhythm may be detected only by inspection, even when it cannot be palpated or auscultated.

2. The techniques are performed in the order given. This order is designed so that subsequent steps reinforce and refine what previous steps have uncovered. In cardiovascular assessment the first step is to inspect the neck vessels and the precordium. Although it is possible that this inspection may offer no clues at all, it may well be that this step would immediately reveal a pathological condition. Succeeding steps would then more precisely define the extent of the problem.

An example of the process of cardiovascular assessment is provided by enlargement of the heart. At inspection one might notice that the client's apex beat had displaced to the left and downward from its location noted on a previous physical examination. This finding alone establishes that enlargement of the heart is present and that the client's condition has therefore worsened. The fol-

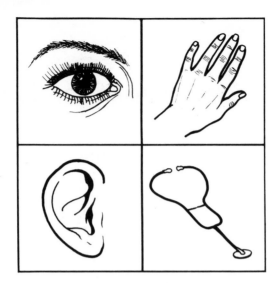

Fig. 4-1. The four assessment tools of cardiovascular assessment. These are the only instruments you will require to adequately assess the heart in an adult. Note that you already own three and that the fourth is simply a hearing aid.

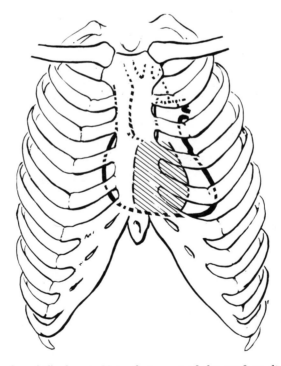

Fig. 4-2. Topography of the heart. Note that most of the surface directly beneath the sternum is composed of right ventricle.

lowing steps would then confirm and elaborate on the cardiomegaly. Palpation would underscore the shifting of the apex beat and adds the refinement of permitting description of the force of the impulse. Until about 20 years ago, percussion would have been used in an attempt to mark the extent of enlargement by mapping out the outer border of the heart. Finally, auscultation would allow the detection of certain sounds correlated with cardiomegaly.

EXERCISE (*see Appendix E for answers*)

1. List the four techniques of modern cardiovascular assessment:

a. _____

b. _____

c. _____

d. _____

MODULE 5

Inspection

Several moments of intense observation should be completed before a hand or a stethoscope is laid on the chest (Fig. 5-1). One must not hurry through this step; it takes time to "warm up" before motions of the chest wall can be correctly identified. Inspection is best done with the client in the supine position, with either the patient lying flat or the head of the bed slightly elevated. It is best to stand at the client's right side for this and all other steps of assessment.

Inspection is performed on the following structures in the order given:
1. Jugular venous pulse (JVP)
2. Carotid arterial pulse
3. Precordium

The venous and arterial pulses will be considered in separate modules, but the above order must always be maintained.

After the neck vessels have been assessed, one then looks for the apex beat, also called the point of maximum impulse (PMI). The apex beat is caused by the heaving up of the left ventricle during contraction, which thrusts the apex against the chest wall. The apex beat is normally not seen in many people (probably more than half the general population) but is most readily seen in individuals with thin chest walls. The apex beat may be difficult to detect in adult females because of the overlying breast tissue, and it is seldom visible in the obese or in persons with a barrel chest caused by chronic pulmonary disease. Inspection can quickly furnish information about two important aspects of assessment concerning the apex beat:(1) location and (2) rate and rhythm.

Location

The PMI is usually found in the fifth left intercostal space (5-LICS) at or just inside the midclavicular line (MCL). To record the location of a normal apex beat, write, "PMI located in 5-LICS inside MCL." If the heart begins to enlarge, the PMI will shift **outward and downward.** The death of portions of the heart muscle, which occurs in myocardial infarction, causes those portions to become hypokinetic and may result in a displacement of the PMI closer to the sternum than usual or even into the fourth left intercostal space (4-LICS).

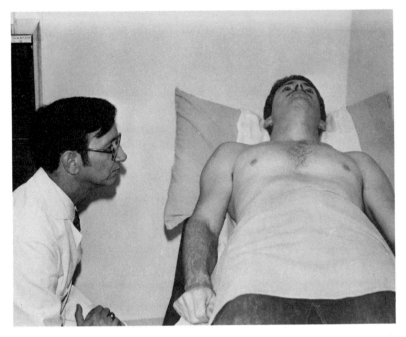

Fig. 5-1. Many abnormal precordial movements are more conspicuous if examiner's gaze is at the level of client's chest.

Rate and rhythm

A brief inspection will permit one to make a rough determination of whether the rate is within normal limits or is abnormally fast (tachycardia) or abnormally slow (bradycardia). Arrhythmias can often be ascertained by inspection. Premature beats can sometimes be seen at the apex, and atrial fibrillation can readily be recognized by apical inspection. In atrial fibrillation the rhythm is totally irregular and the strength of each thrust will vary greatly, with forceful beats interspersed unpredictably between weak ones.

Next, one should look for abnormal movements of the precordium. The four types of abnormal precordial movements are

1. Heaves
2. Lifts
3. Pulsations
4. Retractions

A heave is an abnormally forceful movement of the chest wall around the area of the PMI that is brought about by enlargement of the left ventricle (Fig. 6-3). A heave has a sideward component to its motion. A lift is an anterior (directly forward) movement of the left parasternal area due to enlargement of the right ven-

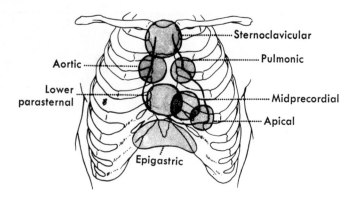

Sternoclavicular

Pulmonic

Aortic

Midprecordial

Lower parasternal

Apical

Epigastric

Fig. 5-2. Areas of chest wall where vibrations are most likely to be detected. (From Hurst, J. W., editor-in-chief: The heart, arteries, and veins, ed. 4, New York, 1978, McGraw-Hill Book Co.)

tricle (Fig. 6-5). An alternate term is a "tap." Although the terminology as given here is preferred, one should be aware that "heave" and "lift" are commonly used interchangeably in everyday parlance.

A pulsation is a movement of the chest wall that is confined to a small site usually in an intercostal space or at the joint of the sternum and one of its attached bones. Normally no pulsations are found on the chest except for the apex beat. Abnormal pulsations can be found at almost any place on the precordium, but the following key areas should be examined (Fig. 5-2):

- Sternoclavicular area
- 2-RICS (aortic)
- 2-LICS (pulmonic)
- Lower parasternal area
- Midprecordial area
- Apex
- Epigastrium

Often the motion of abnormal pulsations can be subtle, and using tangential lighting or inspecting with the eyes at the level of the client's chest helps to define it.

A retraction is an inward motion of either a rib or an intercostal space. There is normally a slight retraction of the intercostal spaces around and near the PMI during contraction of the ventricles (systole). As the heart volume becomes smaller, the inward movement takes place. Any other retractions are always abnormal. Inspection is better for detecting retractions than is palpation.

The finding of abnormal precordial movements probably indicates disease and warrants physician consultation.

EXERCISE *(see Appendix E for answers)*

1. List the correct order for cardiovascular inspection:

   a. _____

   b. _____

   c. _____

2. The PMI is usually found in the _____ LICS just inside the _____ _____ .

3. In cardiac enlargement the PMI shifts _____ and _____ _____ .

4. List the four types of abnormal precordial movements:

   a. _____

   b. _____

   c. _____

   d. _____

5. A directly anterior movement of the area of the chest wall near the lower left sternal border is termed a _____ .

6. A motion of the chest wall in the area of the apex beat that has a sideward component is called a _____ .

7. An inward motion of a rib or intercostal space is known as a _____ .

MODULE 6

Palpation

The main purpose of palpation is to confirm what was found at inspection, but occasionally it will reveal a finding not obtainable by inspection or any other means. Like all other aspects of physical assessment, it is best done with the client in the supine position and the examiner standing at the client's right side.

In addition to the abnormal precordial movements one looks for at inspection, the examiner is also searching for the presence of **thrills** during palpation. Thrills are the purrlike vibrations that accompany some murmurs (Module 27: Murmurs). In addition, one must bear in mind that **all the heart sounds may be palpable.** In fact, extra heart sounds can sometimes be detected by palpation (or inspection) even when they cannot be heard. The proper technique is to rest the flat of the hand lightly on the chest wall. If there is a positive finding, a *little* pressure may possibly allow it to be felt more clearly.

Palpation generally obliterates the JVP but is useful in evaluating the carotid arterial pulse. The carotid artery is palpated by some examiners with a thumb whereas others prefer to use the first two fingers. After the carotid artery has been palpated, the precordium is evaluated, and attention is once again first directed to the PMI. The flat of the hand should be placed directly on the chest wall overlying the spot where the apex was located at inspection (Fig. 6-1). The PMI can then be more precisely localized by using the pad of one fingertip (Fig. 6-2). The apex beat cannot be palpated in a considerable number of normal people.

PALPATION OF THE APEX BEAT

A principal reason one palpates the apex beat is to determine the presence of **left ventricular hypertrophy** (LVH). Palpation is a powerful tool for assessing enlargement or thickening of the left ventricle, and it may well be superior to the ECG or chest x-ray film in its accuracy of detection when performed correctly. There are four characteristics of the apex beat that delineate the extent of LVH: location, size, force, and duration.

Location

As previously mentioned, the PMI can usually be found at or just medial to the midclavicular line (MCL). It is not normally found outside the MCL unless the client has scoliosis or an unusually elevated diaphragm, as might be expected

26

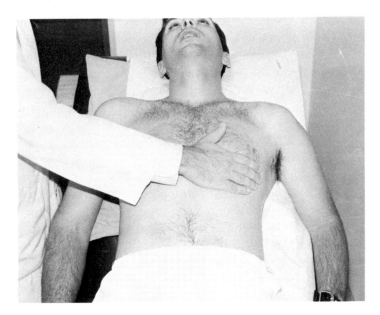

Fig. 6-1. Assessing PMI by palpation. The palm is lightly draped over chest wall.

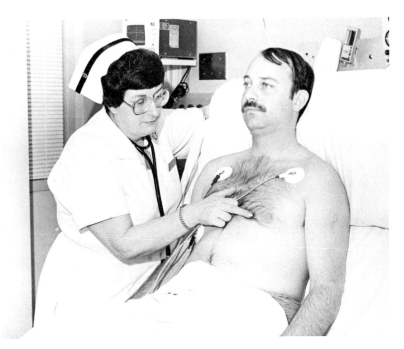

Fig. 6-2. Once the apical beat has been located with the palm as in Fig. 6-1, it is sometimes useful to further delineate the site and characteristics of the PMI by using fleshy pad of one fingertip.

in a pregnant woman. Localizing the apex beat lateral to the MCL should always at least make one suspicious of LVH. In extreme cases of LVH the PMI may be palpated as far as the postaxillary line down to the seventh left intercostal space (7-LICS). **Always palpate the left axillary area** to avoid missing PMIs that have been displaced to the left. Another error to avoid is tilting the client to the left, which could cause the PMI to seem abnormally displaced in an outward direction, giving the appearance of LVH.

Size

The size of the PMI is normally no larger than 2 or 3 cm. Any measurement greater than 3 cm in diameter (size of a quarter) or an apex beat visible in two intercostal spaces is generally abnormal and suggests LVH. However, be wary of the emaciated client, whose PMI may seem abnormally large, leading one to suspect hypertrophy when none is present.

Force

When the heart enlarges, the heart muscle lies closer to the chest wall and the force of the contracting ventricle is more readily perceived. Normally the apex beat presents as a brief tap on the flat of the hand. In LVH the force of the thrust is felt to be greater, and the impulse will "dome up" in the examiner's palm. If the force of the contractions is marked, the impulse will raise the chest wall surrounding the PMI in an outward and sideward direction; this is a heave (Fig. 6-3).

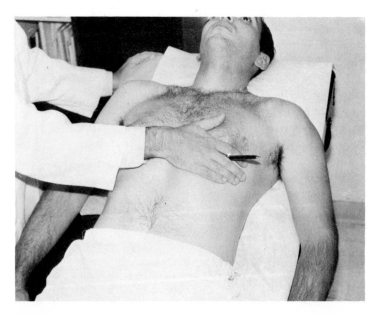

Fig. 6-3. Outward and sideward direction of a heave is indicated by pencil.

Duration

Duration is the most important clue to LVH. The apex beat is normally just a momentary tap that is said to occupy only the first third of systole. As LVH progresses, the duration of the impulse will increase to more than half of systole. The slight tap eventually becomes a steady, sustained swell that lasts throughout the whole of systole. (Means for the timing of systole are discussed in Module 14: The Cardiac Cycle and Assessment.)

PALPATION OF LOWER LEFT STERNAL AREA

Next, place the flat of the examining hand on the lower left parasternal area (Fig. 6-4). Palpation of this area is especially helpful in evaluating for the presence of **right ventricular hypertrophy** (RVH). It will be noted from the diagram of the topography of the heart (Fig. 4-2) that most of the heart tissue directly beneath the sternum is made up of right ventricle. When the right ventricle hypertrophies, a sustained lift of the chest wall adjacent to the sternal border can be felt by the palm during systole (Fig. 6-5). The direction of the lift is directly anterior (Fig. 6-6).

An important type of RVH is **cor pulmonale,** which is enlargment of the right ventricle resulting from chronic pulmonary disease such as emphysema. RVH

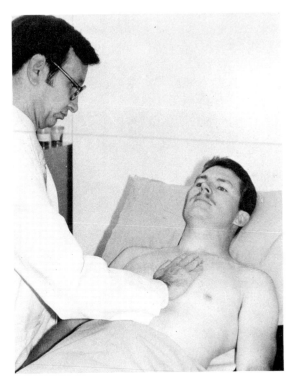

Fig. 6-4. Palpating along left sternal border to detect a lift.

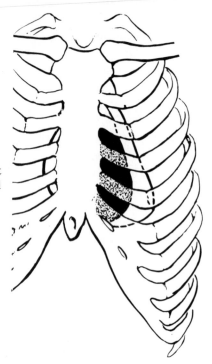

Fig. 6-5. Hypertrophy of right ventricle causes a lift to be felt adjacent to left sternal border. Darkened area represents right ventricle.

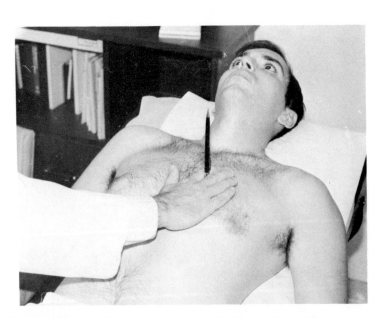

Fig. 6-6. The directly anterior direction of a lift is indicated by the pencil.

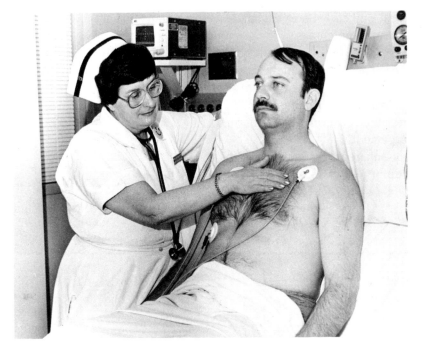

Fig. 6-7. Palpating at base of heart.

generally becomes more difficult to assess as emphysema advances, because the "barreling" of the chest (i.e., the increasing anteroposterior diameter) tends to obscure the characteristic parasternal lift. In such cases it may be possible to detect the RVH by inserting the tips of the first two fingers just under the rib cage to the left of the xiphoid process. The impulse caused by the contraction of the enlarged right ventricle can then be discerned through the fingertips.

PALPATION AT THE BASE

Finally, the examiner places a hand over the base, or upper portion, of the heart at the second right and left interspaces (Fig. 6-7). The hand is used to detect pulsations, thrills and the vibrations of abnormally loud heart sounds which will be discussed later.

SUMMARY

Palpating the three foregoing areas is generally sufficient for the routine cardiovascular examination. If inspection of the neck and entire precordium and palpation of these three areas did not yield positive findings, then one may proceed with the next steps of the examination. If however, there were positive findings, or one has reason to suspect a condition that may produce abnormal motions of the chest wall elsewhere (such as an aortic aneurysm), it may be necessary to palpate surrounding areas of the chest or to probe specific areas with the finger-tips (e.g., in assessing aortic aneurysm one must place the fingertips over the sternoclavicular joints and down into the suprasternal notch [Module 38: Aortic Aneurysm]). One may summarize what one looks for *at each area* during the step of palpation by the mnemonic HEART:

*H*eart sounds (normal and abnormal)

*E*nlargement

*A*bnormal precordial movements

*R*hythm

*T*hrills

If no abnormalities are found at palpation, the precordium is said to be "quiet."

EXERCISE *(see Appendix E for answers)*

1. Locating the PMI lateral to the MCL should alert one to the possibility of

   _____ .

2. In evaluating the PMI, always check the _____ area.

3. A PMI larger than _____ cm is considered abnormal.

4. The most important clue to LVH is the _____ of the apex beat.

5. The surface of the heart directly beneath the precordium is made up mostly of

   _____ .

6. A systolic _____ of the left parasternal area is a sign of right ventricular hypertrophy.

7. In evaluating _____ in persons with barrel chests, insert the tips of two fingers under the left costal margin to pick up RVH.

MODULE 7

Percussion

Percussion is an especially useful tool in assessing the pulmonary and abdominal systems, but it is of no value in direct assessment of the heart. Until approximately two decades ago, percussion was widely employed to demarcate the borders of the heart in an attempt to identify cardiomegaly. In recent years a consensus has grown that this method is ineffective for estimating the size of the heart and that four techniques exist which are superior to percussion for detecting enlargement:

1. X-ray examination
2. Electrocardiography
3. Echocardiography
4. Palpation

Many experts agree that palpation is comparable to the first two techniques for detecting early hypertrophy of the heart and is certainly less costly and time consuming than the third.

The value of percussion in regard to the heart is in evaluating the pulmonary and abdominal sequelae of heart failure. If the left side of the heart fails, pressure is transmitted backward through the pulmonary veins, causing fluid to accumulate in the lungs. In a similar manner, if the right heart fails, pressure "backs up" through the inferior vena cava to the liver, causing fluid to congest this organ and make it swell. Percussion is useful in detecting and measuring the extent of pulmonary and hepatic edema from CHF. It is a simple technique that is easily and quickly applied, and for this reason it will be briefly described.

The basic maneuver utilized in percussion resembles the impatient tapping of a person's fingertips on a tabletop. The main difference is that in percussion a finger from the other hand is interposed into the path of the striking finger so that the interposed finger acts as an anvil.

The purpose of percussion is to determine the composition —whether solid, liquid, or gas filled—of the tissue underneath the area being struck. The principle on which the sonar is based is used in percussion. The blow generates vibrations that enter the underlying tissue and are reflected back, producing a note characteristic of the tissue involved. The denser the tissue, the more the vibrations are damped and the duller is the percussion note. The less dense the tissues, the more hollow sounding the note.

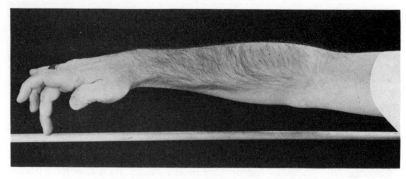

Fig. 7-1. At the start of percussion, the plexor (hammer) finger assumes the form of an arc, and the other fingers are raised away from chest wall.

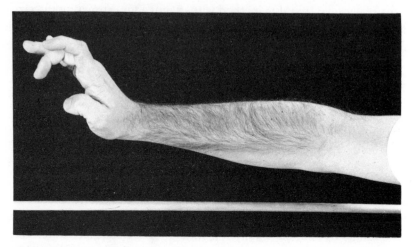

Fig. 7-2. The hand is cocked back at the wrist almost as far as it will go.

The technique is as follows: The two middle fingers are used, one as a hammer (called the plexor) and the other as an anvil (the pleximeter). The fingers of the anvil hand are spread, and the two distal phalanges of the middle finger are then pressed firmly (but not forcefully) against the chest wall. How the plexor hand is held is unimportant. The essential point is that the hammer finger be extended out from the others in the shape of an arc (Fig. 7-1). What one does with the rest of the fingers is of no concern provided they do not contact the chest.

The objective in percussion is to strike the anvil finger a quick, crisp blow with the hammer finger and to deliver each blow with the same amount of force (Fig. 7-2). Avoid pounding or attempting to be lightning quick. The blow is almost entirely the result of snapping the wrist—only a very little forearm motion is used (Fig. 7-3).

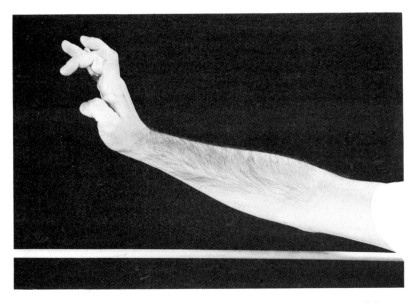

Fig. 7-3. The forearm is raised slightly. At this point, the wrist is snapped downward.

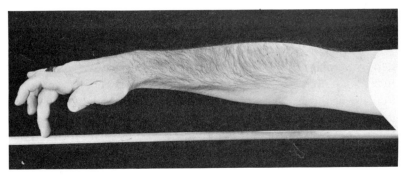

Fig. 7-4. End of percussion blow. Note that the arm is in the same position as at the start of percussion. (Fig. 7-1).

The target is the distal interphalangeal (DIP) joint of the pleximeter finger. The hammer finger is withdrawn the instant the percussion note is generated (Fig. 7-4) because if contact is prolonged, the vibrations will be damped by the very finger that produced them, giving a falsely dull note. Avoid striking the area between the DIP joint and the fingernail, since this tissue is rather sensitive, and examiners who use it tend to unconsciously hedge their percussion blows, producing misleadingly soft notes. (A blow that is too soft may be misinterpreted as being dull.) There are three basic types of percussion notes, and they are described by their pitch or tone (*not* their loudness) as being resonant, dull, or hyperresonant.

Resonant note

A resonant note is produced over the spongy, air-filled tissue of the lungs and is therefore the note that is heard over most of the chest. Percuss your own chest, especially in the areas below the clavicles and the sides of the rib cage, to hear and feel the characteristic resonant note.

Dull note

The dull percussion note is produced when resonance is impaired. It is obtained over tissue that is mostly liquid, such as over a lung base that has filled with fluid (abnormal). In the chest, dullness can be elicited normally only over the areas of the heart and liver (Fig. 7-5). If the quality of resonance is entirely absent from a percussion note (i.e., if the note is maximally dull), it is said to be flat. Flat notes are obtained over structures that are mostly solid, such as the thigh or scapula.

Hyperresonant note

Hyperresonance is the opposite of dullness. Hyperresonant notes are found over tissue that is mostly air filled. The percussion sound "hyperresonates" in the same way that any sound would do so in a large, empty room or a cave, taking on something of a hollow or drum like quality. For example, this kind of note could be elicited by percussing the barrel chest of someone with emphysema. A maximally hyperresonant note is said to be tympanitic. Tympany can normally be elicited only over those spaces on the body that are completely filled with air or gas, such as an area of pneumothorax or a bubble in the stomach or intestines. To hear a tympanitic note, percuss over an empty stomach or a puffed-out cheek.

The two pulmonary manifestations of failure of the left side of the heart are pulmonary edema and pleural effusions. Since both phenomena are gravity dependent, the fluid accumulates at the lowest point. If the client is sitting, therefore, the fluid will pool at the bases of the lungs first and then gradually work its way up to higher lung zones. A dull note can be percussed over such an area of fluid collection. Begin by having the client sit upright and with the shoulders bowed forward, if possible (Fig. 7-6). Percuss the back, starting at the apices of the lungs and working toward the bases. Compare each side for symmetrical resonant percussion notes before moving down to the next level. Percuss at levels that are no more than 4 cm apart. Be especially alert for the presence of dull notes in the area of the lung bases. It may happen that there is a greater accumulation of fluid in one of the lung bases, with less or no fluid in the other, thus giving rise to asymmetrical notes (one dull and the other more resonant). The assessment is more serious the higher that dullness can be percussed in the lung fields.

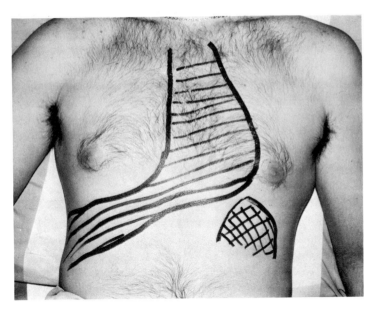

Fig. 7-5. Areas of percussion notes on the normal chest. The area of the diagonal lines represents dullness over heart and liver. The cross-hatched area is tympanitic over gastric air bubble and gas in splenic flexure of colon (this area is variable in size from individual to individual and even from time to time in same individual). Resonant notes are percussed in the remainder of chest.

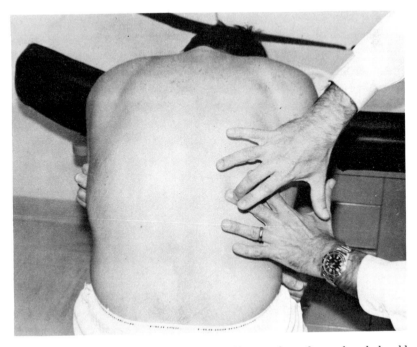

Fig. 7-6. Correct position to percuss the lungs. Client is bent forward and shoulders are drawn together.

The edema of right-sided CHF may also cause the liver to become swollen and enlarged. The liver is percussed in the midclavicular line (MCL) with the client supine. Begin in a resonant area of the lung above the liver and work downward a couple of centimeters at a time until resonance or tympany is again encountered over the abdomen below the rib margin. This point corresponds to the lower edge of the liver and is also marked. The distance between the two marks, the area of liver dullness, normally measures no more than 12 cm in the MCL.

EXERCISE (*see Appendix E for answers*)

1. The most superior technique of physical assessment for detecting cardiomegaly is

   _____.

2. The importance of percussion in relation to the heart is in assessing the pulmonary and

   abdominal sequelae of _____.

3. Describe the percussion note that is produced over the following kinds of tissue:

   a. Fluid-filled: _____

   b. Spongy, air-filled tissue of normal lungs: _____

   c. Hyperinflated lung tissue, as in the client with emphysema: _____

4. Fill in the missing step in the following spectrum:

   Flat → Dull → Resonant → Hyperresonant → _____

5. Failure of the left side of the heart may result in two types of fluid accumulation that produce dull percussion notes over the lung fields:

   a. _____

   b. _____

6. In failure of the right side of the heart, enlargement of the liver is due to

   _____.

7. Normally the area of liver dullness percussed in the MCL measures no more than

   _____ cm.

MODULE 8

Auscultation

Before the nineteenth century, auscultation of the heart was performed by draping a thin cloth over the subject's chest and applying the ear to the cloth. This method was called direct auscultation. Then the Frenchman Laennec discovered the technique of indirect auscultation (as quoted in Hurst, 1978):

> I was consulted in 1816 by a girl who presented the general symptoms of heart disease and in whom palpation and percussion gave little information on account of the patient's obesity. Her age and sex forbade an examination (by direct auscultation). Then I remembered a well-known acoustic fact, that if the ear be applied to one end of a plank, it is easy to hear a pin's scratching at the other end. I conceived the possibility of employing this property of matter in the present case. I took a quire of paper, rolled it very tight, and applied one end of the roll to the precordium; then inclining my ear to the other end, I was surprised and pleased to hear the beating of the heart much more clearly than if I had applied my ear directly to the chest.

Although the stethoscope is indeed a powerful assessment tool, resist the urge to apply this instrument to the chest. Auscultation comes last! If one has performed the previous steps systematically, there may be no need to auscultate in some cases, since no further information would be revealed. (Of course, there are some conditions that are exposed only by auscultation.)

Although it is imperative to listen intently during auscultation, **do not strain.**

Straining inevitably leads to hearing murmurs and other sounds that are not there. Be wary also of the "emperor's new clothes syndrome," which sometimes afflicts beginning auscultators. In this "syndrome," novices "hear" what someone else seemingly more knowledgeable has heard, whether or not it is actually there. This error occurs not only because the "authority" may be mistaken but because some heart sounds are variable, even on a minute-to-minute basis, and what is present on one occasion may be different or even absent on another.

Most examiners find that they are more comfortable if they auscultate from the client's right side. If the client is a woman, both the examiner and client generally find the examination less embarrassing if the auscultator lifts the client's left breast when listening at the apex of the heart. If doing so is difficult for the auscultator because of position or other reasons, the client should be requested to lift the breast.

A serious pitfall in auscultation is failure to eliminate sources of extraneous

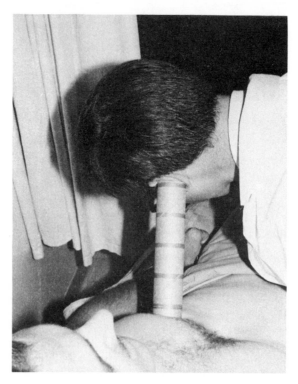

Fig. 8-1. Auscultating with cardboard tube. Sounds from the chest tend to be conducted up rigid, hollow tube rather well. In this instance a tube from a roll of paper towels was used and the normal heart sounds were distinctly heard, although they were moderately faint.

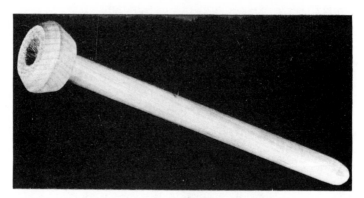

Fig. 8-2. A wooden stethoscope made by my 11-year-old son. Heart sounds are heard with surprising clarity with this device, illustrating the importance of rigidity in the conduction of sound. The stiffer the tubing, the better the transmission of sound. Metal tubing would be the best carrier of sound (impractical), plastic is next best, and rubber comes close behind plastic provided that the rubber is firm.

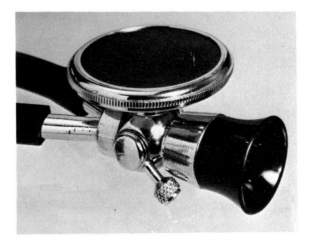

Fig. 8-3. Bowles type of stethoscope. Note the trumpet-shaped bell.

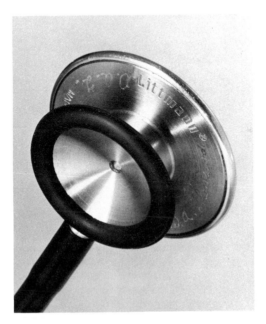

Fig. 8-4. Popular single-tube or Littmann type of stethoscope.

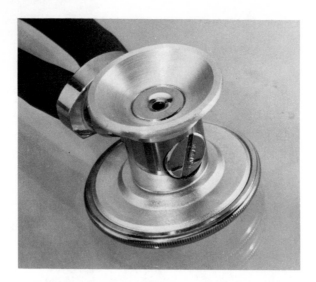

Fig. 8-5. Sprague-Rappaport type of stethoscope.

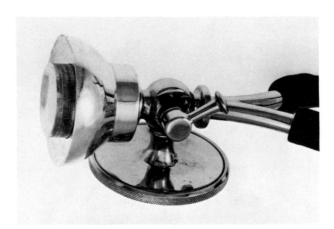

Fig. 8-6. Leatham type of stethoscope. Large, outer bell is excellent for gathering low-frequency sounds in most adults and can be retracted (shown here) to expose a smaller, inner bell that is handy for examining children and adults with thin chest walls.

sound. Not only can extraneous noise mimic some heart sounds, but they may also cover others, so that they are not recognized at all. There are four common sources of extraneous noise:

1. Muscular sounds
2. Respiratory sounds
3. Mechanical sounds
4. Rhetorical sounds

Muscular sounds can be eliminated by first ensuring that the client is warm and comfortable so that shivering is precluded. It is often helpful when one is focusing on a certain heart sound to ask the client to stop breathing for a moment or two so that the distracting sounds of respiration are not present. It is necessary for all doors and windows to be shut, and television sets, air conditioners, and other nonessential machinery should be turned off. Although the "rule of silence" during auscultation has been observed since ancient times, it is interesting how often the rule is violated nowadays. It is especially disregarded during auscultation of the blood pressure, as if this part of physical assessment were somehow less important than other parts. One cannot help but wonder how many instances of systolic hypertension have been missed because those early soft beats were not heard because of continuing conversation by others present. These observations are of considerable practical significance. Silverman (1974) mentions a study in which recordings of heart sounds were played to physicians in a soundproof booth. A recording of ordinary hospital background noise was then played together with the same heart sounds. The heart sounds became audible only when their volume was amplified 12 times!

When one is not sure of a certain sound, it is helpful to close the eyes for a few moments. Another maneuver that sometimes helps in the identification of dubious sounds is to nod the head slowly up and down, with the earpieces in the ear canals, until the sounds come in clearly.

The overall best position of auscultation of the adult client is supine, with the head of the bed slightly elevated (the semirecumbent or semi-Fowler's position). If possible, avoid auscultation with the client lying completely flat or propped at an angle greater than 45°. Auscultation performed only while the client is sitting in the fully upright (high Fowler's) position is unsatisfactory unless circumstances such as acute illness preclude evaluation in a lower position. The client's arms should be at the side, since raising them will decrease the loudness of the heart sounds. If the client has freedom of movement, and if findings in the supine position (or other clinical signs) so indicate, further evaluation may be needed while the client is in the following additional positions:

1. Lying on the left side (**left lateral decubitus** position). If this position is to be used, instruct the client to turn on the left side and use the left arm as a pillow curled beneath the head. The client then drapes the right arm over the side of the right leg. The examiner *uses a footstool* and, if the client is still exhibiting muscular movement, steadies the position by having the client lean backward against the examiner's torso. Further support can be given, if needed, by placement of the examiner's left hand on the client's right shoulder.

2. Sitting and leaning far forward with the breath held in expiration (**seated flexion** position).

The indications for assuming these positions are discussed in modules to follow, which explain the details of the process of auscultation. **In children, it is absolutely necessary to auscultate in both the lying and sitting positions.**

MODULE 9

Arterial pulse

The arterial system is assessed by
1. Blood pressure readings
2. Inspection of the carotid artery
3. Palpation of the arteries
4. Auscultation of the arteries

Many examiners begin cardiovascular assessment by taking the blood pressure and feeling the radial pulse. This approach helps to relax the client, and inspection of the neck and precordium can often be accomplished while the radial pulse is being evaluated.

The arteries that are indispensable for assessment are the carotid, radial, femoral, dorsalis pedis (DP), and posterior tibial (PT). Additional arteries that are accessible and used to corroborate findings are the temporal, brachial, and popliteal. The carotid gives the best impression of the arterial waveform (Fig. 9-1), but it is more convenient to begin with the radial artery.

Always feel the pulses on both sides. One examines for five aspects of the arterial pulse: (1) rate, (2) rhythm, (3) force (also called amplitude), (4) form of the pulse wave, and (5) nature of the arterial wall.

RATE

Some authorities recommend counting the pulse for 30 seconds and multiplying by two to obtain a pulse rate that is adequate for routine purposes. Others state that a period of 15 seconds multiplied by four is sufficient to obtain the approximate heart rate, but in no case should the counting time ever be less than 15 seconds. If an abnormally fast or slow pulse is found, or if an irregularity is present, however, count the pulse for a full minute by auscultation at the cardiac apex to obtain the apical rate (the so-called A rate).

RHYTHM

An irregular pulse must be further described as *regularly irregular* or *irregularly irregular*. The former is most likely caused by a pattern of premature beats that are occurring on a regular basis, whereas the latter is almost certainly the result of atrial fibrillation.

44

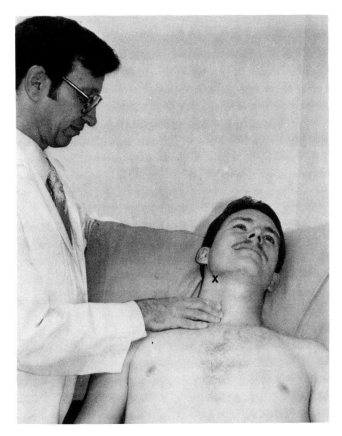

Fig. 9-1. Palpating the carotid artery. Character of pulse wave is best appreciated by using three fingers. Confine palpation to lower half of artery to avoid stimulating carotid sinus body, located where indicated by **X**.

FORCE

Force is recorded on a scale of four, as follows:

  0 = Impalpable
 +1 = Feeble; barely palpable
 +2 = Decreased
 +3 = Full
 +4 = Bounding

Although the finding of a decreased pulse always arouses concern about the possibility of impaired circulation or other disease process, one should bear in mind that it is normal to find a decreased pulse or on occasion even an absent pulse as an individual variation. This is especially true of the popliteal, brachial, and posterior tibial pulses. The probable reason is that pulses are more deeply buried in some people. (Conversely, a few individuals normally have bounding pulses. For example, the radial artery may be so close to the skin that a strong pulsation can be seen at the wrist even when the client is at rest.) Generally the finding of a decreased pulse is not significant, **provided that a more distal pulse is palpable.** In the case of the most distal pulses (radial in the upper extremity, and DP and PT in the lower), decreased or absent pulses bilaterally are sufficiently suspicious that one must search aggressively for other signs of adequate circulation, such as warmth of the part, full motion, lack of paresthesia, and quick filling of the capillary beds in the nails. In addition, it is fortunate that in the foot there are two arterial pulses (DP and PT) that can be used as alternates for checking circulation, for when one is absent the other usually is present (Figs. 9-2 to 9-5).

A finding that is much more significant is **asymmetrical pulses.** Such pulses are nearly always the result of a pathological lesion. To compare for symmetry of the pulses, it is helpful to palpate both sides at the same time, *except* in the case of the carotids. **Never palpate both carotids simultaneously.** Pressing on both carotids in unison may incite hypersensitive carotid sinus bodies to shut down

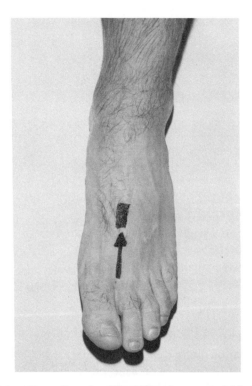

Fig. 9-2. Location of dorsalis pedis pulse. The DP pulse can quickly be located by tracing an imaginary line that follows groove between first and second toes.

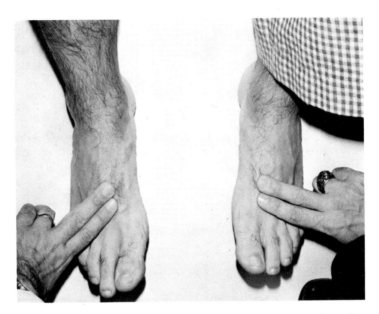

Fig. 9-3. Palpating DP pulse, which is best done with pads of two or three fingers draped over dorsum of each foot. Symmetry of pulses is most quickly and accurately assessed by simultaneous palpation.

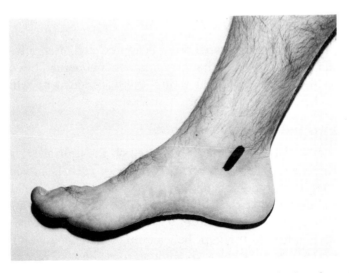

Fig. 9-4. Location of posterior tibialis (PT) pulse. This pulse can be found just behind and slightly below medial malleolus.

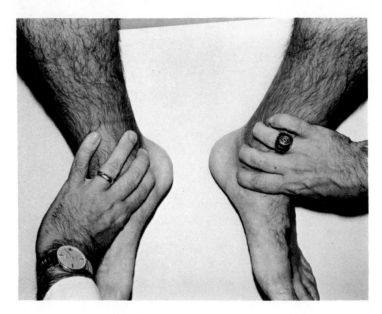

Fig. 9-5. Palpation of the PT pulses.

the heart beat, which may then prove difficult to restart. Persons who are taking **digitalis** preparations are particularly susceptible. When routinely evaluating the carotids, one can avoid carotid sinus stimulation by confining palpation to the **lower half** of the artery. Use the thyroid prominence (Adam's apple) as a landmark, remembering to keep the fingertips below it.

FORM OF THE PULSE WAVE

The shape of the normal arterial pulse is appreciated after only a few pulses have been palpated (Fig. 9-6). Although a number of abnormalities of the arterial pulse have been described in the literature, there are four with which every examiner should be familiar.

Water-hammer pulse (collapsing pulse)

The first name calls attention to what is felt on the upstroke, and the second name describes the downstroke. The water-hammer pulse is a strong, bounding pulse easily detected by the fingers. The water-hammer was a child's toy in Victorian England that consisted of a glass tube several inches long and containing only a vacuum and a small amount of water. When the tube was inverted, the bolus of water plummeted through the vacuum and collided with the bottom of the tube, producing a sharp thud. In addition to rising very quickly, the water-hammer pulse falls away so quickly that it is sometimes called "collapsing." This combination of rapidly rising and falling away imparts a quality to the pulse that has been variously described as jerking, knocking, or slapping.

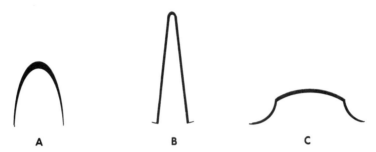

Fig. 9-6. Graph of important arterial pulses that suggest how they are felt by fingertips. **A,** Normal pulse; **B,** water-hammer pulse; **C,** plateau pulse.

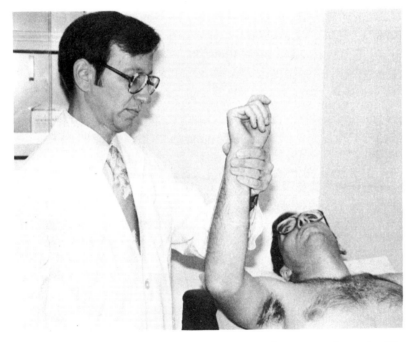

Fig. 9-7. Palpating water-hammer pulse. This maneuver brings out sharp, thudding quality of upstroke and hastens runoff, accentuating collapsing quality of downstroke.

The best method for assessing the pulse is to place the palm over the client's wrist area and raise the client's arm high over the head. This maneuver greatly reduces the normal pulse, but the water-hammer pulse will be conspicuous in this position. In addition, gravity is utilized to assist the "runoff" of the pulse and make its collapsing aspect more evident (Fig. 9-7).

This type of pulse is almost exclusively associated with aortic regurgitation.

Plateau pulse

The plateau pulse is a small, weak pulse, exactly the opposite of the water-hammer pulse. In contrast to the normal pulse, the plateau pulse is slower to rise, seems to maintain itself at a constant level for a moment, and then fades as it falls away. This finding may be detectable only in the carotid arteries and is characteristic of aortic stenosis.

Paradoxical pulse

Actually, "paradoxical pulse" is a misnomer, because there is nothing paradoxical about this pulse at all. Normally the arterial pulsebeat is slightly weaker during inspiration because the heart and great vessels can expand a bit more freely inside the chest cavity, which thus lowers the arterial blood pressure a trifle. The difference between the force of the arterial pulsebeat during inspiration and during expiration is ordinarily so small that it cannot be appreciated by the fingers, but it can usually be detected with a blood pressure cuff. By making careful readings of the systolic blood pressure during both inspiration and expiration, the examiner can observe that the inspiratory pressure is several millimeters of mercury less than the expiratory pressure. Paradoxical pulse is simply an exaggeration of this normal inspiratory decrease in the systolic pressure and is said to exist when the decrease is more than 10 mm Hg. It is commonly associated with conditions that hamper the heart's systolic contractions, such as constrictive pericarditis or pericardial effusion, and with severe asthma and chronic obstructive pulmonary disease (COPD).

Alternating pulse

Alternating pulse is another kind of pulsebeat that is difficult to detect by palpating with the fingers, but it is readily detected with a sphygmomanometer. In alternating pulse the rhythm is regular, and weak beats alternate with strong ones. When the blood pressure cuff is inflated and the pressure slowly lowered, the stronger beats will be heard first. When the pressure of the cuff reaches that of the weaker beats (usually about 10 mm Hg lower), they will become audible and the rate of beats will suddenly double. Alternating pulse is characteristic of severe left-sided heart failure and is a grave sign (Module 37: Congestive Heart Failure).

NATURE OF ARTERIAL WALL

In a young person the walls of all the arteries but the carotids are impalpable except during the systolic pulsations. In later years the process of arteriosclerosis may cause the arteries to become indurated and tortuous, and they are felt as hard cords. It is especially important to assess arteriosclerotic changes in the carotids because of their eventual impact on the brain (as in cerebrovascular accident). Assessment is made by palpation and auscultation. After the carotids are palpated, the diaphragm of the stethoscope should be placed over the arteries. If atherosclerotic plaques on the inside of the arterial walls are disturbing the blood flow, sounds of turbulence called **bruits** can be heard (Module 27: Murmurs). Be wary to avoid pressing at all when auscultating arteries with the diaphragm, because if any artery is sufficiently compressed, turbulence may be produced artificially and **false bruits** will be heard.

EXERCISE *(see Appendix E for answers)*

1. The artery that gives the best impression of the arterial waveform is the

   _____.

2. An arterial pulse felt to be somewhat decreased but not truly weak would be graded

   +_____.

3. Mr. Art Terry is having an evaluation of his left lower extremity. The examiner cannot locate the femoral, popliteal, or PT pulses but does find a DP pulse that is rated +3. These findings indicate that the circulation to the extremity is *(check one)*:
   A. Probably normal
   B. Probably abnormal

4. Some years later Mr. Terry has a cast applied to the left leg, extending from the knee to the ankle. The femoral pulse is graded +4 and the popliteal, PT, and DP pulses are graded 0. The findings are *(check one)*:
   A. Probably normal
   B. Probably abnormal

5. Palpation of both carotid arteries at the same time may result in _____of the heartbeat, especially in a person taking _____.

6. When Ms. Platt is being examined, her peripheral pulses are found to be feeble, and her carotid pulse is noted to be small and prolonged. These findings are characteristic

   of _____.

7. When the difference between the systolic BP during inspiration and during expiration

   is greater than _____ mm Hg, _____ pulse is said to exist.

8. The opposite of plateau pulse is _____ pulse.

9. In an assessment of the nature of the arterial wall, avoid compressing the artery with

   the diaphragm, since compression may produce a false _____.

10. Pericardial effusion may hamper the heart's contractions and cause a

    _____ pulse to appear.

11. The quick, bounding pulse associated with aortic regurgitation is the

    _____ pulse.

12. A poor sign found when the left side of the heart is in severe failure is known as

    _____ pulse.

MODULE 10

Venous pulse

The venous pulse is sometimes called "the window to the right side of the heart." Since all the systemic veins ultimately empty into the right side of the heart (the right atrium specifically), the pressure in the veins is determined to a great extent by the condition of the right heart. Although various veins such as those on the back of the hand or the underside of the tongue have at times been used for a crude evaluation of the venous pulse, the internal jugular vein is favored because its structural arrangement permits accurate determination of the venous pulse pressure at the level of the right atrium.

The internal jugular vein has been referred to as "the manometer of right atrial pressure." Note in Fig. 10-1 that it connects directly to the vena cava, which in turn connects directly to the right atrium. Since there are no valves at any point in this channel, there is a continuous pathway that allows pressure changes in the right atrium to be transmitted up or down this "column" and then detected in the internal jugular vein.

If pressure in the right atrium becomes high, pressure throughout the venous system will rise, and the veins will tend to become engorged or distended. The closer the vein is to the heart, the more likely distention is to be seen. In the internal jugular vein, engorgement first appears at the base of the neck and climbs up toward the earlobe as pressure rises. The distention in the internal jugular vein causes the venous pulsations to become visible, and the pressure in the right atrium can be gauged by measuring the level that the pulsations reach.

What are the causes of elevated pressure in the right atrium? The following phenomena are commonly responsible:

1. *Failure of right ventricle.* This cause of elevated pressure in the right atrium is *always* the first consideration when the venous pulse is elevated. When the right ventricle begins to fail, the blood is not ejected forward into the pulmonary artery effectively, and the pressure from the amount of blood that is left behind in the ventricle backs up into the atrium and then into the neck veins. (See Module 37: Congestive Heart Failure.)

2. *Hyperkinetic circulation.* In this condition the blood simply circulates through the body faster than usual. Hyperkinetic blood flow of course raises the pressure in the other chambers as well as in the right atrium, but the venous

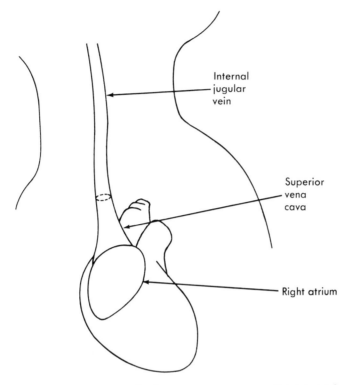

Fig. 10-1. Jugular venous column, which acts as manometer of right atrial pressure. Because there is no impediment in this pathway, there is direct transmission of pressure from right atrium into internal jugular vein.

pulse permits its measurement. Perhaps because hyperkinetic circulation is a generalized phenomenon that occurs so frequently, it is sometimes missed as a factor in venous pulse elevation. The major hyperkinetic states (also termed "high output" states) are associated with the following:

    a. Exercise
    b. Fever
    c. Hyperthyroidism
    d. Pregnancy
    e. Anxiety
    f. Anemia
    g. Stimulant drugs

    3. *Fluid overload.* Perhaps the commonest cause of elevated right atrial pressure in clients with IV lines in place, fluid overload also has a tendency to be overlooked. Whenever a "run-away" IV line is found, the venous pulse should be one of the first parameters to be assessed.

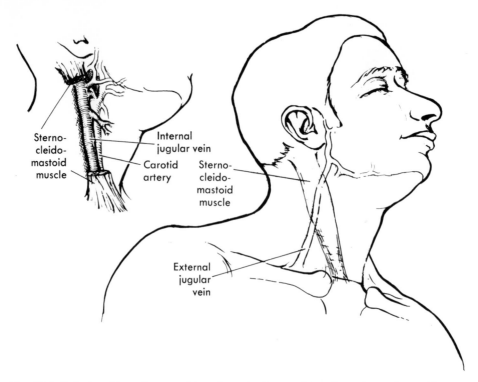

Fig. 10-2. Relationships of external jugular vein, internal jugular vein, and carotid artery. Note especially that the external jugular crosses the outside of the sternocleidomastoid muscle.

4. *Constriction around the heart.* Another condition that tends to elevate the pressure in all four chambers, this constriction can occur with constrictive pericarditis, pericardial effusion, or cardiac tamponade.

5. *Tricuspid valve disease.* If there is narrowing of the valve opening (stenosis), the valve resists the atrium's attempts to empty itself, and increased atrial pressure results. Atrial pressure also rises if the atrium receives extra blood from backward flow across a leaky valve (regurgitation).

The jugular venous pulse is also elevated if there is an obstruction of the superior vena cava, but here the mechanism is not increased right atrial pressure. The venous blood flow from the brain to the heart simply cannot pass the obstruction very well; thus the blood piles up in the internal jugular vein, causing it to engorge.

In an assessment of the venous pulse it is best to disregard the external jugular vein unless for some reason, such as obesity, the internal jugular is not visible. The external jugular has the property of engorging easily and conspicuously with very little provocation, such as breath holding, wearing tight clothing, or twisting the neck. Distention of the internal jugular is more subtle. The inter-

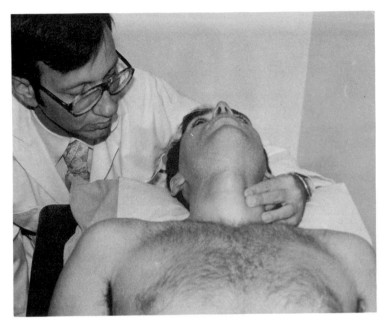

Fig. 10-3. A good way to differentiate between carotid artery pulse and internal jugular pulse is to inspect the right side of the neck while palpating the left. If the pulsation visible on right coincides precisely with palpable carotid pulsation on left, then the visible pulsation must likewise be arterial. On the contrary, if the visible pulsation is venous, the X trough will occur as the carotid pulse reaches its peak.

nal jugular is located under (deep to) the sternocleidomastoid muscle and runs in the same direction along its length (Fig. 10-2). Thus one looks for the internal jugular pulse beginning with the root of the neck just lateral to the sternoclavicular joints and scanning upward along the course of the sternocleidomastoid until finally the earlobe is reached.

The carotid artery runs parallel to the internal jugular vein, which sometimes leads to confusion. Perhaps the easiest way to distinguish the arterial pulse from the venous pulse is to recall that the venous pulse is a low-pressure pulse that is almost never palpable; the carotid pulse, on the other hand, is a high-pressure pulse, and the harder one presses, the clearer this pulse becomes to the fingertips. Thus one can palpate the carotid artery on the left while inspecting the venous pulse on the right (Fig. 10-3). What one looks for is a gentle in-and-out pulsation of the skin and muscle tissue overlying the internal jugular. The carotid pulse, in contrast, has an up-and-down motion. The reason is that in cross section the carotids are circular, whereas the jugulars are elliptical (Fig. 10-4). In addition, the bolus of blood traveling through the arteries is much larger and more discrete than the gentle wave passing through the veins. The arterial

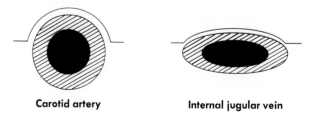

Carotid artery   Internal jugular vein

Fig. 10-4. Cross sections of carotid artery and internal jugular vein. Since the carotid is round, the bolus of blood from each heartbeat traveling through it gives the appearance of an up-and-down motion, whereas the flow through elliptical jugular vein causes an in-and-out motion.

pulse is sharp and quick, wherease the venous pulse more slowly wells outward and inward. The differences between the arterial pulse and the venous pulse are summarized below:

Aspect	Carotid artery	Jugular vein
Form of pulse wave	Single	Double
Palpation	Felt better with increasing pressure	Impalpable
Inspection	Crisp, discrete	Soft, diffuse
Motion	Up-and-down	In-and-out
Respiratory variation	None	Clearer on expiration, fainter on inspiration
Effect of position	None	Lowering head increases, raising head decreases

In a healthy person the internal jugular pulse is seen only when the subject is lying flat. In fact, a good way to begin studying the venous pulse is by inspecting the neck veins of healthy individuals who are completely recumbent. In this position, at least a portion, if not all, of the jugular should be engorged. As the head of the bed is raised, the venous pulse begins to collapse, and the head (top) of the column of venous pulsations can be seen to recede toward the chest. In a healthy subject the pulse will often totally disappear by the time an angle of 15° is reached. From approximately 15° to about 60° there is a gray zone where visible venous pulsations may be normal or abnormal, depending on where the height of the pulsations is measured. Above 60° almost any visible pulsations would be indicative of a high right atrial pressure, since by this point the column of pulsations would normally have fallen below the clavicle. In extreme elevation of right atrial pressure the internal jugular is distended along its entire length, even when the client is in a completely upright position.

Thus, somewhere about midway between lying totally flat and sitting up straight there is a point, in the vast majority of people, where the head of jugular pulsations will appear between the clavicle and the earlobe. Gently lower and raise the head of the bed until this point is found and becomes maximally visible. It will generally be found between 30° and 45°, but always begin by making a preliminary inspection with the client at 45°. Loosen the client's collar and place a small pillow behind the head to relax the sternocleidomastoid muscles. Lift the chin if necessary to remove any wrinkles, and turn the head slightly away from the side that is to be inspected. As with all pulses, examine both sides for symmetry, but for measuring the height of the venous pulse use only the right side, since kinking of the left innominate vein will falsely elevate the jugular pulse on that side. Tangential lighting will accent the venous pulsations and make them clearly visible. If it becomes necessary to use the external jugular for assessment, one can quickly ascertain the highest point of pulsation by compressing the vein with one finger just above the clavicle (Figs. 10-5 and 10-6). Blood coming from the head will rapidly engorge the entire external jugular. When the vein has filled, release the compression and the vein will empty except for "true" distention produced by right atrial pressure. (This maneuver does not work for the internal jugular.)

When the client has been placed at an angle of 45°, a preliminary rough assessment is made by simple inspection before the bed position is altered for the purpose of measurement. At this angle the normal venous pulse will never be visible higher than 1 cm above the clavicle. This spot assessment will then enable the examiner to determine the angle at which the head of the bed should be placed to bring out the venous pulsations. If there are no pulsations, the bed should be lowered. If the right atrial pressure is high, the level of pulsations will be over 1 cm, and if the level of pulsations is very high, the bed may need to be raised. In severe cases the level of pulsations will ascend the sternocleidomastoid until it becomes intracranial, and the earlobe can be seen to pulsate.

The reference point used to measure the venous pulse for recording is the sternal angle (angle of Louis or manubriosternal junction), which is located at the 2-LICS. One must draw two imaginary *horizontal* lines, one at the level of venous pulsations and the other at the level of the sternal angle. The measurement is made in centimeters of the *vertical* distance between the two parallel lines (Fig. 10-7) and is normally not more than 4 cm. *Do not measure directly from the head of pulsations to the sternal angle.* The reason the sternal angle is used as a reference point is that regardless of the position of the head of the bed, the relationship between the two horizontal lines is stable; that is, as the client's position changes, the level of pulsations fluctuates relative to the position of the sternal angle, so that the distance between the two lines is maintained. Nevertheless, the angle of the client's position is always indicated in recording, together with which jugular vein is used for assessment (external or internal). An example of recording is, "The internal jugular pulse is 7 to 8 cm above the sternal angle with client at 45°."

The central venous pressure (CVP) is defined as the pressure at the midpoint

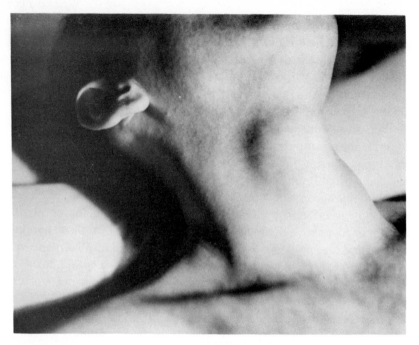

Fig. 10-5. Lighting from the side (tangential lighting) is valuable in defining pulsations of neck vessels. Note that external jugular vein is scarcely visible in this photograph.

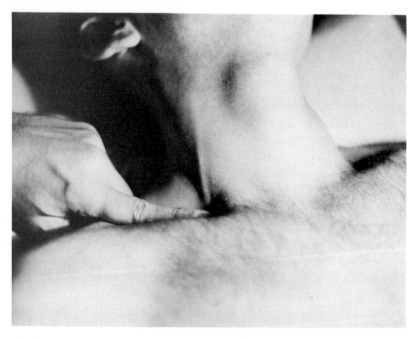

Fig. 10-6. External jugular vein is artificially engorged. This maneuver is helpful in precisely determining the extent of external jugular distention. Finger occludes vein to rapidly fill the vein with blood along its entire length. Then finger is withdrawn and vein is observed as it collapses downward to client's true level of jugular distention.

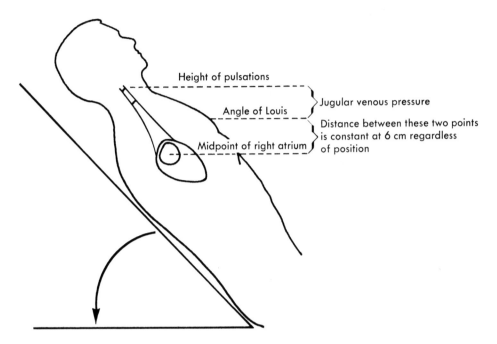

Height of pulsations

Angle of Louis

Midpoint of right atrium

Jugular venous pressure

Distance between these two points is constant at 6 cm regardless of position

Fig. 10-7. The JVP is measured as vertical distance in centimeters between height of internal jugular vein pulsations and angle of Louis. The CVP can be estimated by adding 6 cm to JVP. The head of the bed is elevated at an angle that will best bring out venous pulsations.

of the right atrium. The CVP is usually measured by means of a manometer with a catheter that has been threaded through a peripheral vein until the tip comes to rest at the center of the right atrium. However, before a CVP line is ever inserted, one can estimate the CVP by using the techniques described above. After measuring the jugular venous pulse, add 5 to 6 cm to it for the distance between the sternal angle and the midpoint of the right atrium, which is also constant regardless of position. The result will be reasonably close to the CVP assessment.

The form of the venous pulse wave can also furnish information about events in the right atrium. Careful inspection will show that the venous pulse is double, consisting of two positive (outward) waves, the A and V waves (Fig. 10-8), which are the result of retrograde transmission of pressure changes in the right atrium. The designations of these waves originated because the A wave is due to atrial contraction and the V wave occurs during the time of ventricular contraction. Their appearance approximately coincides with the heart sounds that correspond to atrial and ventricular contraction, that is, the first heart sound for the A wave and the second heart sound for the V wave. (See Modules 16 and 17, which discuss these heart sounds.) Between the two positive waves there appear two negative (inward) waves, or "troughs," called the X and Y descents. Sometimes

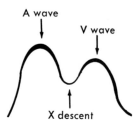

Fig. 10-8. Graph of jugular venous pulse as it appears at inspection. The JVP is seen at root of neck as a "double flicker" of approximately equal waves, with the A wave only slightly more prominent than the V wave.

machines that graphically record the venous pulse can also detect a tiny third positive wave called the C wave, but it can rarely be detected clinically and has no significance for assessment.

What one looks for is a missing or unusually large A or V wave. The venous pulse is normally a "double flicker," with each of the positive waves being of approximately equal prominence. If one of the positive waves is absent, the venous pulse will appear single, which is abnormal. If one of the waves is absent, it almost always is the A wave, and since the A wave is the direct result of atrial contraction, it can be deduced that atrial fibrillation is responsible. Large A waves can be seen if there is resistance to emptying of the right atrium, as in tricuspid stenosis or pulmonary hypertension, or if the atria beat against a closed tricuspid valve, as happens when there is junctional tachycardia or complete heart block. Large V waves are seen whenever there is backward flow in the atria during ventricular contraction, as in tricuspid regurgitation.

Do not spend a great deal of time trying to identify the contour of the venous pulse wave, since this facet of assessment is inherently difficult, especially if the heart rate is fast or the venous pressure is high. One can use the general rule that if much time must be spent searching for an abnormality of the venous wave form, there probably is none, or it will be picked up in some other part of the cardiovascular examination.

EXERCISE *(see Appendix E for answers)*

1. The internal jugular vein is called "the manometer of ＿＿＿＿＿＿＿＿＿ pressure."
2. Which of the following conditions is unlikely to elevate the JVP?
   A. Fluid overload
   B. Right heart failure
   C. Hypotension
   D. Pericardial effusion

3. The ＿＿＿＿＿ wave is produced by contraction of the right atrium.

4. With the client at 45°, spot assessment of the JVP will normally show pulsation no

   higher than _____ cm above the clavicle.
5. Which of the following drugs are unlikely to contribute to an elevated venous pulse?
   A. Propranolol
   B. Caffeine
   C. Amphetamine
   D. Nicotine

6. If the JVP appears single, it is usually because the _____ wave is missing.
7. In atrial fibrillation the atria do not contract effectively and the ventricles contract
   irregularly. Therefore, in this condition, one would expect to see a single venous pulse

   that appears irregularly and that in reality is the _____ wave.

8. If the JVP is elevated, the first consideration is *always* _____.

9. Large A waves may be seen if there is resistance to _____ of the
   right atrium.
10. Ms. V. Ness begins to complain that she has become aware of "something turning
    over inside my chest." To evaluate the significance of these palpitations, the examiner
    makes a complete cardiovascular assessment. After inspection of Ms. Ness's neck, the
    examiner cannot decide whether the visible pulsations are arterial or venous. During
    palpation the felt impulses coincide with the visible impulses. Therefore the pulse

    visible on inspection must be _____.
11. The diffuse in-and-out motion of the JVP is explained in part by the fact that a cross

    section of the internal jugular vein is _____ in shape.

MODULE 11

Using the stethoscope

The stethoscope one chooses should have the following characteristics:
1. Headpiece (Fig. 11-1) should have both diaphragm and bell.
2. Ear tips should fit snugly but comfortably.
3. Tubing should be **thick** and **double.**
4. The shorter the tubing, the better (a length of not more than 30 cm [12 in] is recommended).

The diaphragm of the stethoscope is used to hear sounds of high frequency, whereas the bell is used to pick up the low-frequency sounds. Thus the precordium must be auscultated twice, once with each side of the headpiece.

Most of the sounds generated by the heart are basically high frequency, with the exception of the following, which are the major low-frequency sounds:
1. Third heart sound
2. Fourth heart sound
3. Murmurs of atrioventricular (A-V) valve stenosis

These sounds will be addressed individually later in the text, but suffice it to say at this point that they can be of great significance in assessing a client's condition. Hence one should become proficient in using the stethoscope bell.

The correct way to pick up the high-frequency sounds is to press the diaphragm firmly into the skin. The bell, on the other hand, must be used with the lightest of touches. The edge of the bell must barely make an air seal against the skin. If any further pressure is applied, the skin underneath will be stretched, in effect becoming a diaphragm and thus blocking out the low-frequency sounds. The examiner should auscultate the precordium twice, once with each side of the headpiece. Many of the heart sounds are in the mid range, that is, between high and low frequencies, and will therefore sound slightly different when heard with the bell and diaphragm. One should gain an appreciation of how these two devices modify *all* the heart sounds. Thus one should use the bell not only where low-frequency sounds would be expected to be heard but in other areas of the precordium as well.

There are three basic types of stethoscope: acoustic, magnetic, and electronic. Acoustic stethoscopes, the most frequently encountered kind, allow the sounds from the body to pass to the ear with little alteration. Magnetic and electronic

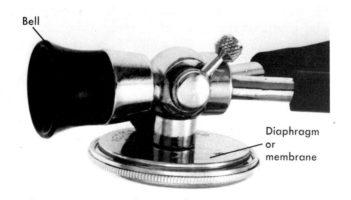

Fig. 11-1. Parts of headpiece of a Bowles type of stethoscope.

stethoscopes interpose mechanical devices in the path of the sound vibrations to alter their intensity (and sometimes their qualities).

Magnetic stethoscopes employ a magnet to amplify the vibrations of the diaphragm to a small extent. Physicists tell us that the magnetic diaphragm does offer a slight advantage in picking up high-frequency sounds over the conventional diaphragm, but stethoscopes with magnetic diaphragms are not popular, probably because of their higher cost and the fact that they must be used with a conventional bell. No magnetic device has ever been shown to be superior to the conventional bell for picking up the low-frequency sounds.

Electronic stethoscopes are expensive instruments that are seldom used in clinical practice. They are so efficient at amplifying body sounds that extraneous noises are often distracting, and the heart sounds are sufficiently distorted that some users accustomed to auscultating with acoustic models have difficulty recognizing the heart sounds.

Of the acoustic stethoscopes, the Sprague-Rappaport enjoys considerable prestige but is not regarded as any better in its acoustic qualities than is the less expensive Bowles. The Littmann is popular for its low cost and easy portability, and although probably adequate for most applications, it is not renowned for superior acoustic properties. The 3M Company, manufacturer of the Littmann, has recently introduced a model called the cardiology stethoscope (not just for cardiologists!) that embodies many of the qualities of the ideal stethoscope.

Whichever instrument is chosen, keep in mind the adage that the most important part of the stethoscope is that which is found between the ear pieces. Even the most sophisticated stethoscope cannot make up for a deficient knowledge base. The choice of an instrument will not matter so much if one knows what to listen for and uses the proper techniques for eliciting the various sounds.

During auscultation of the client with a hairy chest the examiner must ensure that the headpiece is held steady so that no rubbing against the hairs occurs, since the sound produced may resemble **crackles** (also called crepitations or rales), which are signs of abnormal moisture in the lungs (for a description of crackles, see Module 37: Congestive Heart Failure). If the client is extremely hairy, it is a good idea to mat the hair with water so that it lies flat against the skin. Care should be taken to see that the tubes do not rub against the skin or each other, since the rubbing may produce sounds that may be mistaken for **murmurs** or **friction rubs.** It is wise to fasten the tubes together with a clip.

EXERCISE *(see Appendix E for answers)*

1. The diaphragm picks up sounds of _____ frequency.

2. In listening for a third heart sound, the _____ of the stethoscope should be used.

3. Crackles, or sounds heard over the lungs that indicate abnormal moisture in them, are

   simulated by the headpiece's rubbing against _____ .

4. The use of the diaphragm requires _____ pressure.

5. The murmurs of _____ valve stenosis are low-frequency sounds.

6. The edge of the bell must barely make an _____ against the skin.

MODULE 12

Origin of heart sounds

The genesis of the heart sounds has not been determined with absolute certainty. There is no sound produced by the heart whose origin is not debated by scientists at the present time. Nevertheless, recent studies have led to broad agreement on a unified concept for explaining the heart sounds. This view holds that the basic mechanism involved in the generation of the four major heart sounds (the first, second, third, and fourth heart sounds) is abrupt changes in movement of the blood mass inside the heart that set up vibrations in the surrounding structures (chamber walls, valves, great vessels, etc.), and it is these vibrations that are heard as the heart sounds.

In the case of the two normal heart sounds (the first and second heart sounds), the motions of the blood mass are brought about when the heart valves close (Fig. 12-1). Although in the past it was thought that the first and second sounds were actually the vibrations that the valve leaflets made as they slammed shut, it is now believed that these sounds are more likely the result of the vibrations of more-distant structures in response to sudden change in the movement of blood. Whatever their exact origin, however, it is clear that production of the two normal heart sounds is at the very least determined by **closure of the heart valves.** As the valves close, vibrations are emitted that are heard as the familiar lubb-dupp sound of the heart sounds.

The lubb sound has been designated the first heart sound and is abbreviated S_1. The dupp sound is the second heart sound, or S_2. The first sound is determined by the closure of the atrioventricular (A-V) valves (i.e., the mitral and tricuspid valves), and the second sound is brought about through closure of the semilunar valves (i.e., the aortic and pulmonic valves).

Systole is the contraction of the ventricles, and events that occur during this period can be heard during auscultation in the interval between S_1 and S_2. *Diastole* is the period of relaxation and filling of the ventricles, and diastolic occurrences can be heard between S_2 and S_1.

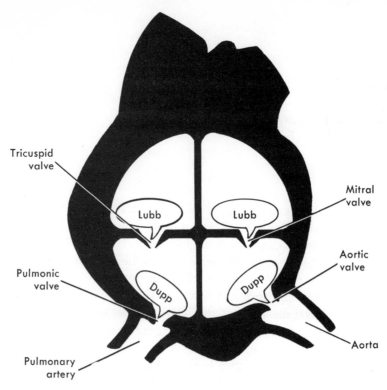

Fig. 12-1. Diagram of the heart. Determining event in production of the two normal heart sounds is closure of heart valves. All the valves, except the mitral, or bicuspid, valve, are composed of three leaflets. The location of the **mitral** valve on the **left** side of the heart can be recalled by the following mnemonic: "The bishop of Heartville wears a **mitred** hat and is **never right**."

EXERCISE *(see Appendix E for answers)*

1. The unified concept for the origin of heart sounds holds that they are vibrations of cardiac structures surrounding points of abrupt change in the movement of the

   _____ .

2. The name of the lubb sound is the _____ .

3. The abbreviation for the dupp sound is _____ .

4. The motions of the blood that generate the two normal heart sounds are associated with

   _____ of the heart valves.

5. The period between the first and second sound is termed _____ .

6. The closure of the _____ valves coincides with S_1.

7. Diastole is the period of relaxation and _____ of the ventricles.

8. The second heart sound is determined by the closure of the _____ valves.

MODULE 13

Auscultatory areas

The four classic or primary areas for cardiac auscultation are shown in Fig. 13-1. Each area corresponds to one of the heart's four valves and is the location on the precordium where the sounds produced by the valve in question are *frequently* the loudest. Thus the sounds produced by the aortic valve will often be heard best in the aortic area, which is located in the second intercostal space (2-ICS) next to the right sternal border. The pulmonic area is located opposite the aortic area in the 2-ICS near the left edge of the sternum. The tricuspid area is found lower down the left sternal edge at the fifth intercostal space. The mitral area is also in the 5-LICS at the cardiac apex. A little rhyme as given by Sherman and Fields (1974) is helpful in committing these locations to memory:

> Aortic right, pulmonic left,
> Tricuspid's 'neath the sternum;
> Mitral's at the apex beat—
> This is how we learn 'em.

There are two important points to note about the classic auscultatory areas: (1) They are *not* located directly over the valves for which they are named. (2) Although sounds originating at a certain valve are *frequently* heard best at the auscultatory area bearing the name of that valve, there are numerous instances in which a sound produced by a valve may be loudest at some distance from the primary area. Probably the foremost example of this second point is the aortic valve, in which murmurs produced by this valve may be heard best in some cases at Erb's point (see following discussion), in other individuals at the lower left sternal border, and in still other individuals, even at the apex or in the neck.

Besides the four classic areas, there are two other major auscultatory areas: Erb's point and the lower left sternal border.

Erb's point

Erb's point is located in the 3-ICS close to the left sternal edge. It is also referred to as the **secondary aortic area,** because some murmurs originating at the aortic valve are so often loudest here. In addition, sounds generated by the pulmonic valve (such as a split second heart sound) may occasionally be heard best here instead of over the primary pulmonic area.

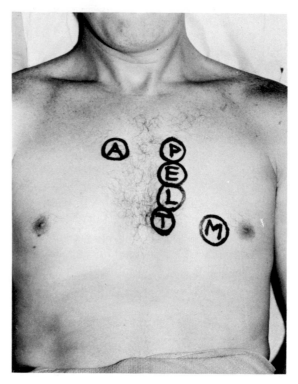

Fig. 13-1. The primary auscultatory areas. *A*, Aortic area; *P*, Pulmonic area; *E*, Erb's point; *L*, lower left sternal border; *T*, tricuspid area; *M*, mitral area.

Lower left sternal border (LLSB)

The LLSB is the area in and around the 4-LICS adjacent to the sternum. It is a good spot to listen for aortic murmurs and friction rubs. In addition, sounds produced by the tricuspid valve (such as a split first heart sound) may at times be transmitted to this area better than to the classic tricuspid area.

Summary

Thus it can be seen that there are six areas that form a chain stretching from the aortic area down the entire left sternal border and across the 5-LICS to the apex beat. However, one must not confine auscultation to the points on this chain but rather must use them only as starting points. Remember that the **entire precordium** is being evaluated and that, in addition, there are times when the neck, abdomen, and back should be auscultated for proper assessment of the heart.

EXERCISE *(see Appendix E for answers)*

1. The mitral area is located at the point of ⎯⎯⎯⎯⎯⎯⎯⎯⎯⎯⎯.

2. Erb's point is also referred to as the ⎯⎯⎯⎯⎯⎯⎯⎯⎯⎯⎯ area.

3. The area just to the left of the sternal border in the 2-ICS is the ⎯⎯⎯⎯⎯⎯⎯⎯⎯⎯⎯ area.

4. "Tricuspid's 'neath the ⎯⎯⎯⎯⎯⎯⎯⎯⎯."

5. The aortic area is found in the ⎯⎯⎯⎯⎯⎯⎯⎯⎯ intercostal space near the ⎯⎯⎯⎯⎯⎯⎯⎯ sternal edge.

6. The apex beat locates sounds produced by the ⎯⎯⎯⎯⎯⎯⎯⎯⎯ valve.

7. Sounds produced by the pulmonic valve may on occasion be louder at ⎯⎯⎯⎯⎯⎯⎯⎯⎯ point than at the classic pulmonic site.

8. In some individuals, sounds produced by the tricuspid valve can be heard better at the ⎯⎯⎯⎯⎯⎯⎯⎯⎯ than at the primary tricuspid area.

MODULE 14

The cardiac cycle and assessment

In auscultating, one should concentrate on each of the four components of the cardiac cycle (Fig. 14-1) in turn:

1. First heart sound
2. Second heart sound
3. Systole
4. Diastole

Even if a certain sound is immediately obvious after the stethoscope is placed on the chest, temporarily block it out and proceed systematically through the cardiac cycle. One's attention should be focused on each component in the order listed above, and concentration should not be shifted to the next component until the sounds of the component at hand have been identified and their characteristics and loudness have been appreciated for a brief moment. This procedure should be carried out in each of the areas one wishes to auscultate. This will probably be relatively easy in most cases because only S_1 and S_2 will be identified.

Thus a complete cardiovascular assessment will involve listening for each of the four components in the six major auscultatory areas, and then listening in other areas of the precordium depending on what one finds in the primary areas and on other clinical clues that may be evident. For instance, if a murmur is encountered, one will want to listen in nearly all areas of the chest in all directions and over the neck to see whether the murmur radiates there. A murmur may also radiate to the axilla or even to the back. In the client with emphysema who has a barrel chest, heart sounds may not be transmitted well to the precordium (they are usually faint or muffled) and may be heard better by listening over the epigastrium.

Personal preference largely determines at which end of the chain of auscultatory areas one begins. Some examiners prefer to start in the aortic area, since it is here that the second heart sound is almost always louder than the first heart sound, and thus the heart sounds are easily identified. Others prefer to listen first at the mitral area with both bell and diaphragm before proceeding to other areas, since many clues for assessment (such as the low-frequency sounds) may be immediately apparent in this area.

It is usually not difficult to identify the components of the cardiac cycle when the heart rate is slow, since systole is noticeably shorter than diastole. However,

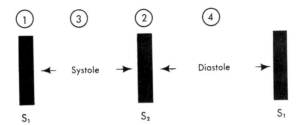

Fig. 14-1. Components of cardiac cycle. The order in which they are listened to is indicated by circled numbers. Note that diastole is a bit longer than systole (at a heart rate of 75, five eighths of cycle is diastole).

as the heart rate increases, the length of diastole shortens until it is nearly equal to systole, making it more difficult to differentiate S_1 from S_2. With practice, one learns to distinguish S_1 and S_2, even at fast rates, simply by their sound characteristics, much as a master learns to recognize his dog by the sound of its bark. In case of doubt one can perform the following three maneuvers to differentiate the two heart sounds and thus time the events of the cardiac cycle:

1. *Auscultate at aortic area.* As already mentioned, S_2 is almost always the loudest of the two sounds here.

2. *Palpate the apex beat.* The apical pulsation taps the palm as S_1 occurs. (Unfortunately, the apex beat is not palpable in many normal people.)

3. *Palpate the carotid arterial pulse.* The upstroke of the carotid pulse occurs at the same time that S_1 is heard. Palpate your own pulse to learn how it feels. (The radial pulse is too far from the heart to be dependable for timing.) It is well to develop the habit of palpating the **lower half** of the carotid artery to avoid pressure on a possibly hypersensitive carotid sinus.

Once the components of the cardiac cycle have been identified, a good technique to avoid "losing" them and having to start all over again is to inch the stethoscope from one area to another rather than making large jumps across the precordium. This technique is especially valuable for revealing the incremental changes in the characteristics of the heart sounds as they travel through the chest.

EXERCISE (*see Appendix E for answers*)

1. The order of listening for the components of the cardiac cycle is as follows:
   a. S_1
   b. S_2

   c. _____

   d. _____

2. As the heart rate increases, _____ becomes shorter.

3. The _____ of the carotid pulse is coincident with S_1.

4. In someone with a barrel chest the heart sounds may be heard best over the

   _____ .

5. The lower portion of the carotid artery is pressed to avoid stimulating the

   _____ .

6. List the three maneuvers for differentiating S_1 and S_2:

   a. _____

   b. _____

   c. _____

7. The first heart sound is heard just as the _____ pulsation taps the palm.

MODULE 15

Heart sound principles

The following are some important principles to keep in mind while reading succeeding modules:

1. Left-sided heart events precede right-sided heart events.
2. Right-sided heart noises are heard best as the right heart becomes engorged with blood during inspiration, thus bringing the right heart into closer contact with the chest wall. Left-sided heart noises are heard best in expiration, when the volume of lung tissue that confines the apex is smallest, thus permitting the left chambers to rise up closer to the precordium.
3. Heart sounds may be conducted through the chest in such a way that they can sometimes be heard best at some distance from their primary auscultatory areas, or from where they are produced.
4. Different tissues alter the conduction of heart sounds (listed in decreasing order of efficiency of conduction).
   a. Liquid (may increase the audibility of the heart sound, although a large accumulation may conduct sound away from its site of production so efficiently that it may be dulled by dissipation)
   b. Bone (good conductor of heart sounds, so that certain noises may even be heard over the skull or at the elbow)
   c. Muscle
   d. Fat
   e. Air-filled (lung) tissues
5. The loudness of heart sounds is decreased by various factors.
   a. Decreased force of contraction
   b. Increased thickness of the chest wall
   c. Increased amount of air in chest cavity (e.g., emphysema, pneumothorax)
   d. Increased fluid around the heart, as in pericardial effusion (see 4a, above; also, if large, may constrict the heart and decrease the force of contraction, as in cardiac tamponade)
6. The loudness of heart sounds can be increased by bringing the structures that produce them closer to the chest wall. Thus sounds produced by the aorta can often be increased by leaning the client far forward so that the

aorta falls against the anterior chest wall, and sounds heard at the apex can be made louder by turning the client to the left side.

7. The sternal edges seem to act as natural channels for the conduction of heart sounds, and vibrations produced in nearby areas are frequently heard better here than in the primary auscultatory areas.

8. Some heart noises that are basically high frequency may become low frequency if their volume is low (e.g., the murmur of pulmonic stenosis) and thus may be audible only with the bell of the stethoscope.

EXERCISE *(see Appendix E for answers)*

1. Closure of the _____ semilunar valve occurs before closure of the _____ semilunar valve.

2. Right-sided heart sounds are heard best in _____ .

3. Rearrange in order of decreasing efficiency of conduction:

   a. fat: _____

   b. bone: _____

   c. air-filled tissues: _____

   d. liquid: _____

   e. muscle: _____

4. In cardiac tamponade the liquid would cause the normal heart sounds to be heard *(louder/fainter)*.

5. You are auscultating a client and hear a murmur whose origin you have narrowed down to either the mitral or tricuspid valve. As you continue to listen, you notice that the murmur becomes louder with inspiration. This tells you that its origin must be the _____ valve.

MODULE 16

First heart sound

The first heart sound (Fig. 16-1) is loudest near the apex of the heart. It is usually the loudest of the two heart sounds at the apex, but there are too many individuals who normally have a louder second sound at the apex to make this generalization dependable for identification of the heart sounds. (Distinguishing the heart sounds is discussed in Module 14: The Cardiac Cycle and Assessment.) S_1 is lower in pitch, duller, and slightly longer than S_2. Listen to your own heart with the stethoscope to see how S_1 becomes louder as the apex is approached and how it fades as the stethoscope is moved toward the base. Compare the first and second sounds to see whether you can appreciate the generally duller quality of S_1 throughout the precordium.

The first sound is produced by the closure of the A-V valves at the beginning of systole. Since the left ventricle is so much larger and more powerful than the right, the force exerted by the blood in the left ventricle to slam the mitral valve shut is greater than the force exerted by the blood in the right ventricle to close the tricuspid valve. Thus the major part of S_1 is produced by the mitral valve, and the tricuspid contributes only a small portion to the total first sound. This explains why S_1 tends to reach maximum intensity (loudness) in the mitral area (apex). Verify this fact on your own chest by comparing the loudness of S_1 at both the tricuspid and mitral areas.

S_1 is made up of two components: the mitral sound (M_1), produced by the closure of the mitral valve, and the tricuspid sound (T_1), produced by the closure of the tricuspid leaflets. As noted above, M_1 is the more intense component of S_1, and it generally drowns out the weaker T_1 over most areas of the precordium. In fact, the tricuspid sound is so soft that it can usually be heard only over the tricuspid area, and even here M_1 is almost always louder than T_1. Sometimes both mitral and tricuspid valves close precisely at the same moment, producing a single first heart sound, whereas at other times there will be a slight difference in the closure of the two valves, producing an audible separation between the two components. When there is an interval between M_1 and T_1 that can be detected by the ear, the first sound is said to be split.

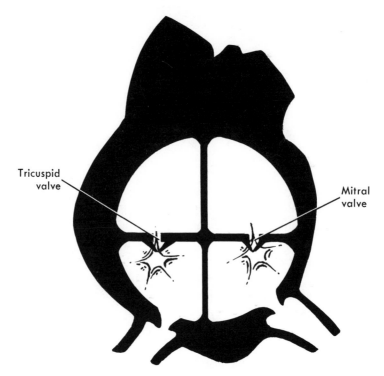

Fig. 16-1. First heart sound is produced by closing of atrioventricular (A-V) valves during contraction of ventricles.

EXERCISE *(see Appendix E for answers)*

1. The area of dominance of S_1 (where it is likely to be the loudest of the two normal heart sounds) is at the _____ .

2. S_1 is *(duller/sharper)* than S_2.

3. S_1 is produced by the closure of the _____ valves at the beginning of _____ .

4. S_1 is made up of two components: _____ and _____ .

5. Of the two components, _____ is the louder; thus the first heart sound tends to be loudest at the _____ area.

6. The best place to hear a split S_1 can be reasoned through as follows:
   a. Auscultating a split S_1 means hearing both components.
   b. The softer component is T_1.
   c. Splitting can best be picked up over the area where the softer component is heard.

   Therefore the best place to hear splitting of S_1 is in the _____ area.

MODULE 17

Second heart sound

The second heart sound (Fig. 17-1) is sometimes called the key to cardiac auscultation. It has earned this title because so many diseases give evidence of their presence by causing characteristic alterations of this sound. Thus it would be well to become familiar with the "bark" of this sound before proceeding. Listen again to your own heart, focusing on the second sound. Listen in various areas of the precordium but concentrate on the base of the heart, where S_2 is heard loudest.

Note that throughout the chest S_2 is of somewhat higher pitch than S_1 and is shorter and snappier than S_1. Once this sharper quality of S_2 is appreciated, the duller sound of S_1 becomes more apparent. As you listen, faintly whispering the words "dull-sharp" as S_1 and S_2 occur will help to establish these qualities in your mind. Note also that the second sound is generally the more dominant of the two heart sounds; that is, S_2 is heard to be louder than S_1 in most areas of the chest. The area of dominance of S_2 is centered at the base and spreads out widely, so that S_2 overshadows S_1 over most of the precordium. Slowly inch your stethoscope away from the heart in several directions and observe how S_1 tends to fade away before S_2. The area of dominance of S_1 is limited and is centered about the apex. Although S_1 is usually the louder of the two sounds in the apical area, the dominance of S_2 is such that in some individuals it may be louder even at this location. Conversely, an S_1 louder than an S_2 at the base is almost certainly an abnormally loud first sound.

The great arteries of the heart, the aorta and the pulmonary artery, house the sources of the second sound, namely the two semilunar valves. As each of these valves snap shut, they generate vibrations that form the two components of S_2: the aortic sound (A_2) and the pulmonic sound (P_2). The aortic component is primarily responsible for the second heart sound and tends to overpower the softer pulmonic sound. In fact, of the four components that make up the two normal heart sounds, A_2 is by far the most intense (loudest), and for this reason S_2 is almost always louder than S_1 in the aortic area. P_2 is usually so soft that it is not likely to be heard beyond the pulmonic area, but A_2 travels well over the entire chest and is audible in almost any location. A_2 and P_2 may occur at nearly the same instant and be heard as a single sound, or they may be separated by various intervals. If these intervals are audible, S_2 is then said to be split.

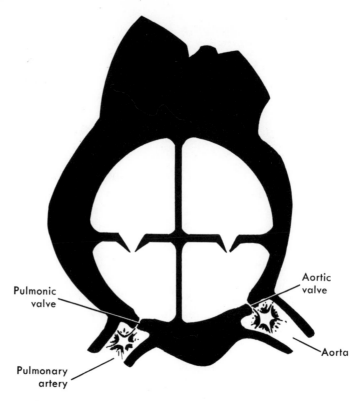

Fig. 17-1. Second heart sound is produced as semilunar valves close. Ventricles have just begun to relax, and these valves snap shut to prevent blood that has been pumped out into systemic circulation and lungs from pouring backward into ventricles.

EXERCISE (*see Appendix E for answers*)

1. S_2 is loudest at the _____ of the heart.
2. S_2 is (*duller/sharper*) than S_1.
3. Select the areas of the chest where S_2 may normally be louder than S_1:
   A. Aortic
   B. Pulmonic
   C. Tricuspid
   D. Mitral
4. The great arteries house the source of the second heart sound, namely, the _____ valves.
5. S_2 is made up of two components: _____ and _____.
6. The major part of the second sound is produced by the _____ component.

7. Of the four components that make up the two normal heart sounds, _____ is by far the most powerful, which explains why S_2 is almost always louder than S_1 in the

   _____ area.

8. The area where splitting of S_2 can be heard is reasoned through as follows:
   a. One must be able to hear both components of the split S_2.
   b. The weaker component is P_2.
   c. Splitting is best detected where the weaker component can be heard.

   Therefore, one can hear splitting of S_2 over the _____ area.

9. An S_1 louder than S_2 at the _____ of the heart is almost certainly an abnormal finding.

MODULE 18

Splitting of heart sounds

So many variables impinge on the contraction of the heart chambers that it is not common for a valve on one side of the heart to close at exactly the same instant as its counterpart on the opposite side; thus there is often some slight separation of the two components of a heart sound (Fig. 18-1). However, if this separation is 0.02 second or less, the human ear perceives the components as a single sound. When the interval exceeds 0.02 second, the ear becomes capable of distinguishing the components as separate.

At the range of 0.02 to 0.04 second it is acknowledged that the difference, although subtle, *is* possible to hear. At this range the crisp single sound begins to become blunted or blurred, and one does not usually hear a distinct **gap** between the two components. A rough analogy can be drawn by saying the word "spit" aloud several times and then saying a few repetitions of the word "split" (try it). Notice how adding the letter *l* to the word "spit" imparted a bounce, which suggests how a heart sound is heard when it is narrowly split. Other terms for this range are "fine" splitting and "close" splitting. A useful rule of thumb is that if one is not sure whether one or two sounds are being heard, a split heart sound in the range of narrow splitting is probably being heard.

At intervals greater than 0.04 second, splitting produces a clearly audible gap, so that two separate sounds are heard. When the space between the two components becomes audible, splitting that is normally wide is said to occur. The upper limit of this normal splitting is 0.07 second. This interval can be approximated by pronouncing the letter "P" two times, as quickly as possible. The interval between the two Ps will be remarkably close to 0.07 second. A sound heard beyond this limit has to be an *abnormally* wide split sound or an extra heart sound.

In summary:

> 0.00 to 0.02 sec = Single heart sound
> 0.02 to 0.04 sec = Narrow splitting
> 0.04 to 0.06 sec = (Normally) wide splitting
> >0.07 sec = (Abnormally) wide splitting or extra sound

It is not uncommon for the beginning auscultator to apply the stethoscope to the chest and, hearing three distinct thumps, to be puzzled about their identities. In this circumstance one is frequently able to readily identify one of the sounds

Fig. 18-1. Models of split heart sounds. Here each heart sound is just barely split. Relative loudness of components is suggested by height of columns. For example, in S_2, the aortic component is normally louder than the pulmonic component.

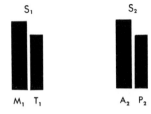

but is not certain whether the other two are (1) a heart sound that is split or (2) an unsplit (single) heart sound plus an extra sound. This dilemma can be resolved by pausing for a moment to evaluate the two unidentified "thumps" on the basis of quality, location, and timing.

Quality

In split sounds the two components are relatively similar to each other in pitch, loudness, and duration. If there is a single heart sound plus an extra heart sound, the two thumps will differ significantly in one or more of these parameters. For example, an opening snap (Module 34: Mitral Stenosis) is distinctly higher in pitch than either the first or second sound.

Location

As you read succeeding modules, take note of the sites where splitting of the heart sound is heard and where the various extra sounds are heard. It will be seen that splitting is not generally heard in those locations where extra sounds are commonly found.

Timing

In splitting, the timing of the two components is relatively close (usually below 0.06 second), whereas extra heart sounds tend to be more distant from the heart sounds they accompany. Perhaps the easiest extra sound to time is the third heart sound, which follows S_2 by about 0.14 second, or approximately double the gap of the widest normal splitting.

EXERCISE (see Appendix E for answers)

1. A blurred or blunted heart sound is in the range of _____ splitting.
2. The upper limit of normal splitting can be approximated by pronouncing the letter

   _____ twice, as quickly as possible.
3. If a heart sound is heard as crisply single, the interval between the two components

   must be less than _____ second(s).
4. A distinctly audible gap of 0.05 second between the components of a heart sound indicates *(normally/abnormally)* wide splitting.

MODULE 19

Splitting of first heart sound

In healthy hearts the closure of the mitral and tricuspid valves usually occurs within 0.03-second of each other; thus it can be anticipated that the first sound will be heard as single in the majority of normal people. Occasional narrow splitting may be found as a normal variation, but normal wide splitting of S_1 is unusual. In fact, normal wide splitting is so infrequent that whenever one believes that a split S_1 is being heard, one is much more likely to be hearing a single first sound plus an extra sound. The additional sound will almost always be one of the following:

1. A fourth heart sound (occurs just before S_1)
2. An early systolic click (occurs just after S_1)

In the normal heart the left ventricle begins to contract slightly ahead of the right, so that mitral valve closure (M_1) precedes closure of the tricuspid valve (T_1). This sequence is in keeping with the principle that left-sided cardiac events occur before right-sided events. However, although the sequence of M_1 followed by T_1 can be seen on the phonocardiogram, the two components occur so nearly simultaneously that for the most part they are heard as single by the ear. When normal (also called physiological) splitting can be heard, it is audible only where the weaker component (T_1) of the split first sound is audible, namely, in the tricuspid area. (In some persons, however, T_1 may be conducted up the left sternal edge, so that it may be heard best somewhat higher than the tricuspid area.)

Normal fine splitting of S_1 is most often heard in adolescents and young adults. The degree of splitting (how wide apart M_1 and T_1 are) does not vary with respiration in some people, whereas in others the splitting is slightly wider in inspiration, and in still others is wider in expiration. Thus with S_1 there is no consistent relationship of splitting to the respiratory cycle.

In the first heart sound, any splitting wider than closely split is likely to be pathological (if the sound is indeed split and the examiner is not detecting an additional sound). The most common pathological splitting of S_1 is due to **right bundle branch block** (RBBB) (Fig. 19-2). In RBBB there is a lesion in the right bundle branch pathway that interferes with the transmission of the electrical impulse down that branch (while the left branch conducts normally). Thus the right branch fires later and the contraction of the right ventricle is delayed. The

82

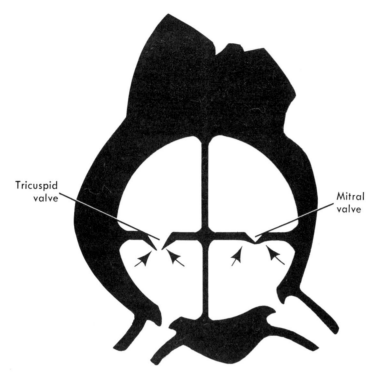

Fig. 19-1. Mitral valve normally closes slightly before tricuspid valve.

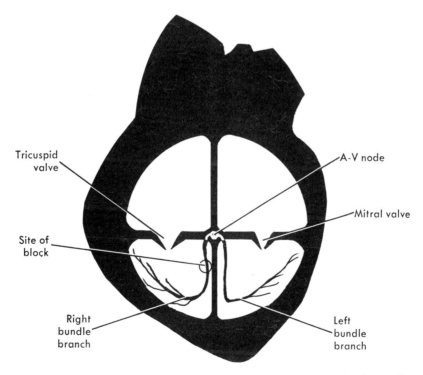

Fig. 19-2. Right bundle branch block (RBBB). Lesion is designated by the small circle.

result is that closure of the tricuspid valve (T_1) lags markedly behind that of the mitral valve (M_1), creating a **wide** (interval more than 0.04 second), **loud** split. Although there are a few other causes, think first of RBBB whenever pathological splitting of S_1 is heard.

EXERCISE (*see Appendix E for answers*)

1. Normal wide splitting of S_1 is so uncommon that whenever it seems to be present, the auscultator should consider the possibility that there is an additional sound as well as a single first sound. List the possible additional sounds:

   a. _____

   b. _____

2. Check which of the following statements is true:
   A. S_1 is ordinarily split in inspiration.
   B. S_1 is ordinarily split in expiration.
   C. S_1 does not display consistent respiratory variation.

3. The most common cause of a pathologically (abnormally wide) split S_1 is

   _____ .

MODULE 20

Splitting of second heart sound

A split S_2 of 0.03 to 0.07 second is a normal finding in **inspiration.** In fact, in most healthy people under the age of 50 years, a split S_2 in inspiration is the rule. The best place to hear this splitting is near the pulmonic area, where the weaker P_2 component is loudest. The heart sounds at this location during inspiration can be represented by the lubb-dlupp sound. As can be seen from Fig. 20-1, A_2, the most dominant of the heart sound components, can be heard well over most of

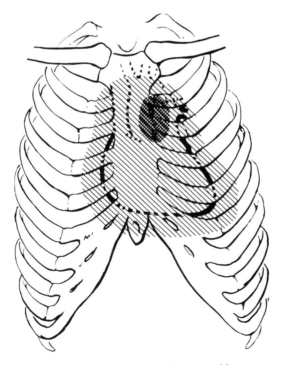

Fig. 20-1. Areas of audibility of the components of the second heart sound. Cross-hatched area = area of A_2; stippled area = area of P_2. A_2 is the most dominant of all the heart sound components and travels widely throughout the chest. P_2 is considerably weaker, and its limited area of transmission is centered about the second intercostal space next to the left edge of the sternum. Thus it is at the pulmonic area where both components of S_2 can normally be heard during inspiration.

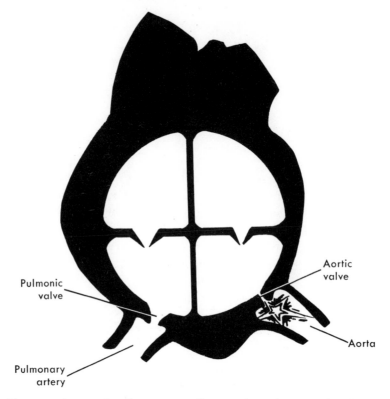

Pulmonic
valve

Aortic
valve

Aorta

Pulmonary
artery

Fig. 20-2. Aortic valve closure normally precedes pulmonic valve closure.

the precordium, whereas the audibility of the softer P_2 is confined to a locality close to the pulmonic area. Thus it is unlikely that splitting will be heard at any site other than the pulmonic area (although individual anatomical variations in some persons may conduct P_2 down the left sternal edge, causing splitting to be heard best at Erb's point), and if it is heard at other sites, it is distinctly abnormal or else indicates an additional sound.

Since left-sided heart events precede right-sided ones, A_2 occurs before P_2 (Fig. 20-2). This is true even in expiration, although during this time the sounds are separated so slightly that they are heard as a single sound. During inspiration the negative pressure inside the chest draws blood into the right side of the heart, filling and distending it so that it takes longer for the right ventricle to contract and "empty" itself than during expiration. Thus pulmonic valve closure (P_2) lags noticeably behind aortic valve closure (A_2). In addition, expanding the lungs causes *less* blood to enter the left side of the heart than when the chest is quiet, which shortens the time of left ventricular contraction and brings on A_2 slightly earlier. The net result is an audibly split second sound during inspiration (Fig. 20-3). During expiration, A_2 and P_2 normally fuse, so that a single sound is heard. S_2 is often single in both inspiration and expiration in elderly people.

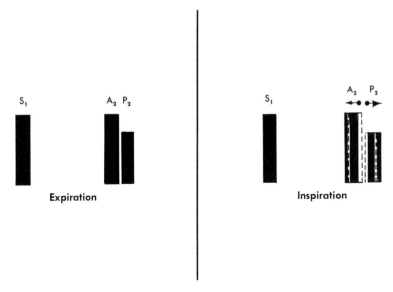

Fig. 20-3. Effect of inspiration on second heart sound. When the chest is quiet in expiration, A_2 and P_2 are so close together that they are heard as a single sound (in the left side of figure the relationship of A_2 to P_2 is exaggerated to the level of narrow splitting for purposes of illustration, but in reality the two sounds would overlap each other slightly). When the subject breathes in, changes within the chest take place, as described in the text, that further widen the intervals between the two components; thus, audible splitting can be detected. Dotted lines represent positions of A_2 and P_2 in expiration, as depicted on left side of figure.

Normally, then, S_2 can be expected to split on inspiration and become single on expiration. In fact, a split S_2 in **expiration is always abnormal** and in every instance calls for physician consultation. The only exception in which expiratory splitting of S_2 is not abnormal occurs in some healthy children and young adults who may have a split S_2 during expiration in the **recumbent** position that becomes single during standing or sitting. This fact is important because many young people have been thought to have an **atrial septal defect** after having been auscultated only while lying down. Therefore, when evaluating an expiratory split of S_2, do not fail to have the client assume a fully upright position!

One of the most common causes of a split S_2 in expiration is also the most common cause of an abnormally split S_1: RBBB. (See Fig. 19-2.) Here the mechanism is the same as for the pathologically split S_1, except that the delayed contraction of the right ventricle results in a retardation in this instance of pulmonic valve closure, so that P_2 occurs markedly after A_2. Since the interval present during expiration is also subject to the normal effect of inspiration as described above, it can be heard to widen further when the client breathes in.

In **left bundle branch block** (LBBB) the reverse occurs. The impulse travel-

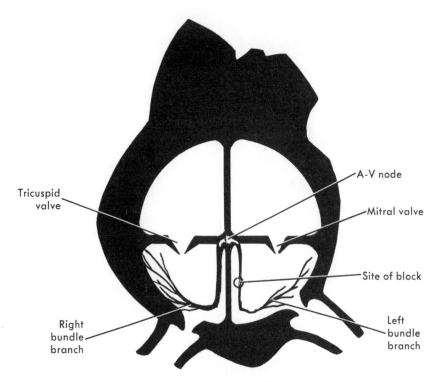

Fig. 20-4. Left bundle branch block (LBBB). In LBBB, the right ventricle contracts before the left when the chest is quiet in expiration; thus P_2 precedes A_2, and an audible split is heard. The effect of inspiration on the second sound causes the P_2 to merge into the A_2, which results in a single sound. This sequence of split S_2 in expiration and single S_2 in inspiration is exactly the reverse of normal. Small circle indicates lesion.

ing down the left branch is retarded, delaying contraction of the left ventricle and in turn delaying A_2 until well after P_2 has occurred (Fig. 20-4). The result is an audible splitting of S_2 during expiration. During inspiration P_2 moves in its usual direction (to refresh yourself on this point, see Fig. 20-3), but in LBBB it merges with the delayed A_2. The position of A_2 is steady in LBBB because A_2 is produced by defective electrical conduction, whereas P_2 ebbs and flows like the tide, gently flowing away from A_2 during expiration and washing back to A_2 with each inspiration (Fig. 20-5). Notice that this splitting of the second sound in expiration and single sound of S_2 in inspiration is exactly the reverse of normal and hence is termed **reverse** or **paradoxical splitting** of S_2.

A good way to gain an appreciation of reversed splitting of S_2, if the opportunity presents itself, is to auscultate someone with an artificial pacemaker in which the electrode contacts the endocardium of the right ventricle (the most frequent location). A pacemaker so implanted produces **mechanically-caused LBBB,** that is, it produces an LBBB pattern on the cardiac monitor and, in addi-

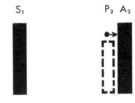

Fig. 20-5. Effect of inspiration on second heart sound in LBBB. Dotted lines represent position of P_2 during expiration. Thus, in inspiration, P_2 and A_2 fuse, resulting in a single sound.

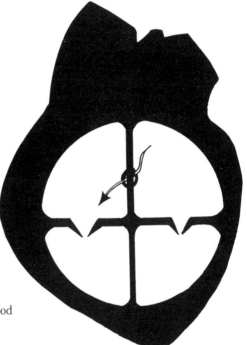

Fig. 20-6. Atrial septal defect (ASD). Blood flows through hole in direction of arrow.

tion, produces the auscultatory finding of LBBB, namely, paradoxical splitting. Place the stethoscope on the pulmonic area and, if the pacemaker is a demand model, observe the monitor for the appearance of branch block patterns; the splitting will be heard simultaneously.

In **atrial septal defect** (ASD) there is an opening in the wall separating the atria that is present at birth (Fig. 20-6). This opening causes the two atria to communicate; thus in effect they become **one chamber.** ASD is an important condition because it is the most common congenital cardiac malformation in adults and is often asymptomatic until the client reaches middle age and begins to experience the early dyspneic symptoms of congestive heart failure. Early detection of this condition is to be emphasized, since corrective surgery is more successful when the client is young. The earliest clue in the child or adult is frequently the presence of expiratory splitting of the second sound, even with the client sitting up straight.

It is important to understand the mechanism that produces the splitting of S_2 in ASD. There is a left-to-right shunt through the septal defect so that the right side of the heart receives extra blood, causing a prolonged emptying time of the right ventricle that gives rise to a delayed P_2 (similar to that discussed in RBBB, which, incidentally, commonly accompanies ASD). Since this split is usually 0.05 second or greater, a distinct **wide** splitting is heard, and an identical gap is heard in inspiration; that is, the interval of the splitting is the same in both expiration and inspiration. This lack of respiratory variation in the split is termed **fixed** splitting and occurs because the normal effect of inspiration on S_2 (review Fig. 20-3) is canceled out by the free communication between the atria. This normal effect of inspiration on S_2 is dependent on an intact interatrial septum; without this effect the atria act as a single reservoir and behave in inspiration just as they would in expiration. In ASD, then, each atrium feeds the same amount of blood to its corresponding ventricle throughout the respiratory cycle, and since the relationship of A_2 to P_2 is maintained, the splitting is fixed, or unchanging. In summary, the hallmark of ASD is **wide, fixed** splitting of the second heart sound.

The mechanisms of production of the two major splitting abnormalities can be recalled by the mnemonic **fix it right,** which indicates that fixed splitting is caused by a lag in the ventricular emptying time of the right side of the heart. The other major abnormality, reverse splitting, is the result of such a lag on the "reverse" (left) side.

When listening for splitting in the pulmonic area, one should compare the loudness of the second sound's components, A_2 and P_2 (Fig. 20-7). In all adults and many children the general rule is that "$A_2 > P_2$" (A_2 is louder than P_2). In a child, however, especially a small child, one can often expect P_2 to be louder, since the pulmonary artery is relatively larger in many children and is closer to the chest wall. In a normal adult, A_2 is always the louder sound because the aorta is larger and has higher pressure in it. Normal changes in the arterial beds that raise the arterial pressure with increasing age also cause A_2 to become louder as one grows older. In known cases of systemic hypertension or arteriosclerosis of the aorta, A_2 becomes considerably more intense than in the normal individual. Since both of these conditions elevate the pressure in the aorta, the aortic valve is slammed shut with greater force than usual, giving off a loud A_2.

Listen for splitting of S_2 in your own pulmonic area and compare A_2 and P_2. If you are healthy, A_2 will be louder than P_2 (or at least of equal loudness). If P_2 is louder, it almost certainly is pathological and points to an elevated pressure in the pulmonary artery (pulmonary hypertension), much the same way that an elevated pressure in the aorta intensifies A_2. The most common cause of an abnormally high pressure in the pulmonary artery is **cor pulmonale;** it should be called to mind whenever a loud P_2 is heard (Module 40: Pulmonary Hypertension). Cor pulmonale, which is enlargement of the right side of the heart secondary to lung

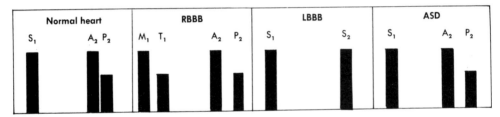

S₂ in inspiration

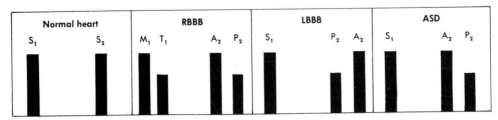

S₂ in expiration

Fig. 20-7. Important variations of second heart sound compared in inspiration and expiration.

disease, is often associated with right-sided heart failure (Module 37: Congestive Heart Failure). The accentuated P_2 of elevated pulmonary artery pressure can sometimes be palpated in the pulmonic area. The finding of "$P_2 > A_2$" (P_2 louder than A_2) can be important and warrants physician referral. Since cor pulmonale is caused by lung disease, a thorough pulmonary assessment is also in order.

In summary:

Abnormally loud $A_2 \rightarrow$ Aortic/Arterial disease
Abnormally loud $P_2 \rightarrow$ Pulmonary heart disease

Comparing A_2 and P_2 for loudness does *not* mean comparing the relative loudness of the second sound in the aortic and pulmonic areas. Rather, one listens for splitting in the pulmonic area, and the assessment of $A_2 > P_2$ or $P_2 > A_2$ should be based on what is found in the pulmonic area alone. Switching the stethoscope back and forth between the aortic and pulmonic areas to comment on the loudness of the dupp sounds in the two locations may be misleading because what is heard in the pulmonic area may be mostly (or even totally) the result of aortic valve closure (A_2). However, if S_2 auscultated in the pulmonic area is louder than S_2 heard in the aortic area, the reason is probably that the pulmonic component (P_2) happens to be unusually loud. This can be verified only by "gluing" the stethoscope to the pulmonic area for a few moments and listening for the split as the client breathes in (it will be heard unless the S_2 is truly single).

A final word of caution about splitting of the second sound: ensure that the client maintains *quiet, continuous* breathing. Respiratory variations in splitting may not be discernible if the breath is held or is not rhythmical. An excellent way to bring out splitting of S_2 and other sounds that display respiratory variation has been described by O'Neal-Humphries (1978) and is called **cycled respiration.** With one hand holding the stethoscope on the client's chest, hold out your other hand in front of you and have the client breathe in as you raise your hand and breathe out as you lower it. This method enables the examiner to know the phase of respiration even with the eyes closed, to listen to an extra cardiac cycle or two in each phase, and to increase venous return to the heart slightly so that certain sounds are louder.

EXERCISE *(see Appendix E for answers)*

1. Fill in the blanks:

    a. Loud $A_2 \rightarrow$ _____ disease

    b. Loud $P_2 \rightarrow$ _____ disease

2. To best hear splitting of S_2, ensure that the client maintains _____,

    _____ breathing.

3. Fixed splitting of S_2 is caused by a delay in the emptying time of the _____ ventricle, whereas reverse splitting is caused by a similar lag in the emptying of the

    _____ ventricle.

4. The most common cause of an abnormally high pulmonary artery pressure (pulmonary hypertension) is _____ .

5. A split S_2 in _____ is always abnormal. However, before recording

    this finding, ensure that the client is auscultated in a fully _____ position.

6. The splitting abnormality heard in ASD is _____ splitting.

7. A _____ S_2 is normal in elderly people throughout the respiratory cycle.

8. One of the most common causes of expiratory splitting of S_2 is also the most common

    cause of an abnormally split S_1, namely, _____ .

9. In children and adults through middle age a split of S_2 in _____ is normal.

10. Splitting of S_2 is best heard in the _____ area or Erb's point.

11. LBBB produces a _____ S_2 in inspiration and a _____ S_2 in

    expiration; for this reason this splitting pattern is termed _____ splitting.

MODULE 21

Third heart sound

A third heart sound (S_3) can be heard in some individuals early in diastole about 0.12 to 0.16 second after S_2 (Fig. 21-1). When the events of the cardiac cycle are timed, S_3 is heard to occur just after collapse of the carotid pulse.

As with the other heart sounds, the origin of S_3 is not precisely certain, but since S_3 occurs during the phase of diastole in which the ventricles are rapidly filling with blood, it is thought that the sound is generated by vibrations when the rush of blood into the ventricles is abruptly halted by ventricular walls that have lost some of their elasticity (Fig. 21-2). For this reason, S_3 is sometimes referred to as the ventricular sound. It has been noted that when S_3 is audible, it gives a triple rhythm that some have fancied as sounding like galloping hoofbeats, particularly when the heart rate is fast, and thus the term "ventricular gallop" is also encountered.

The third sound is best heard at the apex of the left ventricle (i.e., at the mitral area) and since it is a sound of **low pitch,** can be best picked up by the **bell** or the ear applied directly to the chest (Figs. 21-3 and 21-4). It sounds like a soft thud, and the rhythm of the two normal heart sounds plus S_3 is suggested by the phrase "lubb-dupp-uh." The third sound is often faint and requires a period of concentrated listening in the area of the apex before it becomes audible. Listen especially closely during expiration, since the S_3 arises from the left side of the heart and is thus heard best during the expiratory phase of the respiratory cycle. Many an S_3 has been missed because the bell was applied and the heart listened to for only three or four beats. The third sound may not appear in all cardiac cycles, being present in some but not in others.

An S_3 can be found in as many as one third of healthy children and teenagers and can normally be found in some young adults (below the age of 30 years), especially those with a thin chest. In this age group a third sound is considered to be physiological (normal) if there are no other abnormal findings on physical examination and if the client is symptom free. In an adult over 30 years of age an S_3 is considered to be potentially pathological and requires consultation with a physician if not previously known. This course of action is recommended even with pregnant women, the majority of whom develop an audible S_3 by the thirtieth week of pregnancy.

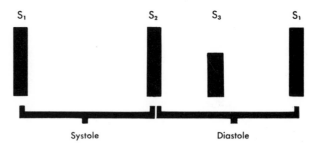

Fig. 21-1. The third heart sound occurs about a third of the way through diastole.

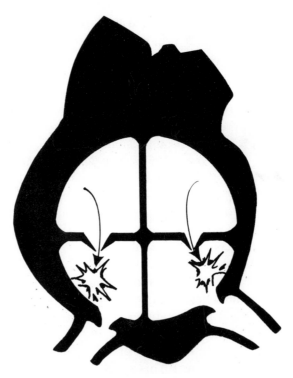

Fig. 21-2. The third heart sound is generated by the collision of columns of blood with the walls of the ventricles during the phase of rapid filling in early diastole.

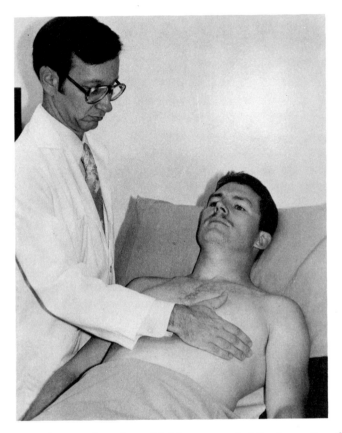

Fig. 21-3. Palpating the apex beat for a third heart sound. After inspecting the lower left hemithorax for the presence of a visible S_3, the palm is used to localize the apex beat and feel for a palpable third sound. If an S_3 cannot be detected by these means, the PMI indicates the site where one then uses the stethoscope to listen for this sound, as shown in Fig. 21-4.

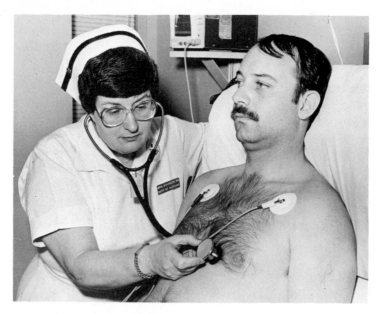

Fig. 21-4. If an S_3 cannot be detected by using the palm of the hand (Fig. 21-3), the PMI indicates the site where one then uses the stethoscope to listen for this sound.

Any condition that hinders the free movement of the ventricular walls can give rise to an S_3, but the usual cause is **heart failure.** In CHF the wall of the ventricle hypertrophies and loses its compliance (stretchiness or elastic quality), sending forth a third sound that becomes louder as the disease advances.

Although the majority of third heart sounds are left-sided (arise from the left ventricle), an occasional right-sided third sound can be found. An S_3 generated in the right ventricle is heard to the right of the apex close to the lower sternal border (tricuspid area) and should be especially looked for in clients with COPD, who may develop right-sided heart failure (cor pulmonale). Besides the location, another point of differentiation is that, like all sounds originating in the right side of the heart, the right-sided S_3 can be heard louder during *inspiration* and at times may be heard over the neck veins as the client breathes in.

Two other conditions commonly associated with an S_3 are mitral regurgitation (MR) and constrictive pericarditis. In the latter the sac surrounding the heart (pericardium) constricts the entire heart, occasioning a loud S_3 known as the "pericardial knock." Although its occurrence in these two entities does not necessarily imply heart failure, it must be emphasized that the prime importance of the appearance of an S_3 is as an indicator of CHF. Since almost any type of heart disease may terminate in failure, it is essential that whenever a client is identified as having a cardiac condition, the examiner should *carefully search for* an S_3 around the apex. The third sound is the only clinical sign that reflects the state of the myocardium itself, and it may be the **first and only sign** that the heart muscle is decompensating. An S_3 is thus an early sign of heart failure, frequently occurring before *any other* sign appears, including pulmonary signs such as crackles.

Inspection and palpation should always be done before auscultation because these operations help to localize the point for auscultation (i.e., the apex beat) and also because an S_3 is sometimes inaudible but can be seen or felt as an extra bounce on the downstroke of the apical pulsation. This bump on the apex beat can be magnified so that its motion is more apparent during inspection by balancing the midpoint of a tongue depressor, broomstraw, or similar object directly on the PMI and fastening it with a thin strip of tape.

A maneuver to help clarify an S_3 is to have the client assume the **left lateral decubitus** (lying on the left side) position. This brings the left ventricle into closer contact with the chest wall. Ensure that the client is steady and comfortable in this position to eliminate muscle noises, and then palpate before auscultating to locate the new PMI.

The third heart sound is accentuated by any **hyperkinetic circulatory state.** The major hyperkinetic states are listed in Module 10: Venous Pulse. If blood circulates in the body faster than normal, the rush of blood into the ventricles and its subsequent collision with the relatively stiffer ventricle walls are greater, accentuating the S_3. A convenient method of increasing the circulation that all but the most ill clients can tolerate is to have the client squeeze the examiner's fingers (sustained handgrip).

EXERCISE (*see Appendix E for answers*)

1. The third heart sound is heard during the phase of diastole in which the ventricles are

   rapidly _____ with blood.

2. Since S_3 is a sound of low frequency, it is best picked up by using the _____ of the stethoscope.

3. S_3 is heard at the _____ of the left ventricle.

4. Cor pulmonale is likely to produce a _____ S_3.

5. The usual cause of an S_3 is _____.

6. Check those clients in whom the detection of an S_3 is probably abnormal:
   A. A 35-year-old man
   B. A 25-year-old pregnant woman
   C. A 65-year-old woman
   D. A 12-year-old girl

7. The third sound may be the _____ and _____ sign of CHF.

8. An S_3 that is heard best at the tricuspid area and that grows louder on inspiration and becomes audible over the neck veins as the client breathes in is *(left-sided/right-sided)*.

9. If a faint S_3 is heard, it can be made louder by turning the client to the

   _____ position.

10. A third sound can be accentuated by any _____ circulatory state.

11. Another term for S_3 is the _____ sound.

12. An isolated finding of an S_3 in a child is considered to be _____ .

13. The S_3 is heard in early _____ .

14. A "pericardial _____" is actually a kind of S_3.

MODULE 22

Fourth heart sound

The contraction of the atria normally produces a sound of such low pitch and faintness that it cannot usually be detected except by the phonocardiograph, but it is commonly made audible by cardiovascular disease. This sound is the fourth heart sound (S_4), also called the atrial sound or, at fast heart rates, the atrial gallop. It is generally the softest of the heart sounds and resembles a gentle thud or a faint footstep on a carpet. It occurs in late diastole (Fig. 22-1), immediately before S_1, when the contraction of the atria kicks extra blood into the filling ventricles, and (like S_3) it becomes audible when there is reduced ventricular wall compliance (Fig. 22-2).

Although S_4 has its origin in the contraction of the atria, the sound is not produced by the motion of the atrial walls themselves but rather by the impact of columns of blood with the stiffened walls of the ventricles, which is the reason it is heard best at the apex. Like S_3, it is detected with the bell of the stethoscope and is accentuated in the left lateral decubitus position. It can often be seen or palpated as a bump, or shoulder, on the upstroke of the apical beat, even when it cannot be heard, and its motion can be made more conspicuous by the "tongue depressor maneuver" described in the previous module. When the events of the cardiac cycle are timed, since S_1 is simultaneous with the upstroke of the carotid pulse, S_4 can be detected just before the carotid upstroke begins. During auscultation the rhythm of "$S_4 + S_1 + S_2$" can be simulated by the phrase "tuh-lubb-dupp." Hyperkinetic states tend to increase S_4's loudness. (For a review of these states, see Module 10: Venous Pulse.)

Already some similarities of S_4 and S_3 can be seen, since they both

1. Are diastolic (S_3 early; S_4 late)
2. Arise in the ventricles
3. Occur during filling of the ventricles
4. Result from decreased compliance of ventricular walls
5. Are heard best with the bell
6. Are louder in the left lateral decubitus position
7. Are louder in hyperkinetic states

As can be seen from Fig. 22-1, S_4 occurs so late in diastole that it comes very near to S_1. It approaches S_1 so closely, in fact, that its presence is easily confused

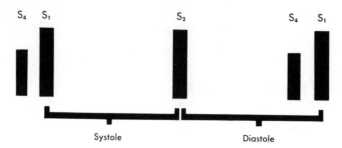

Fig. 22-1. The fourth heart sound is heard in late diastole.

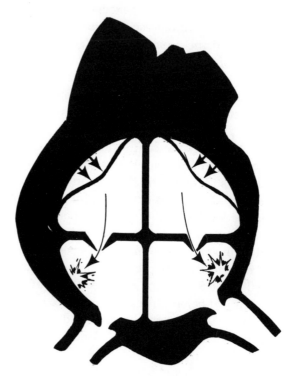

Fig. 22-2. The fourth heart sound is produced by the contraction of the atria, which propels more blood into the already filling ventricles.

with a split S_1. Recall, however, that splitting of the first sound is heard where the softer T_1 component is audible, namely, in the tricuspid area, and that the S_4 is usually heard at the apex (unless it is a right-sided S_4, which indeed *is* heard best close to the tricuspid area). Therefore what is "heard" at the apex as a split S_1 is most likely to be, in reality, an S_4 followed closely by an S_1.

The S_4 can be heard in many healthy persons over 50 years of age. It has been said that what makes an S_4 normal or abnormal is "the company it keeps," that is, the presence or absence of other clinical findings of heart disease (this criterion also applies to an S_3 in an individual under the age of 30 years). When heart disease is present, S_4 becomes louder as the severity of the disease increases. Detection of an S_4 in anyone below the age of 50 years, or in anyone over this age if there are any other findings of cardiovascular disease, warrants physician consultation.

The forms of heart disease that most often produce a fourth heart sound are LVH, RVH, and ischemic heart disease.

LVH

One of the earliest indicators of hypertrophy is the S_4, and it is more than occasionally heard before the other visual or palpable signs become evident. The most common cause of an S_4 is **systemic hypertension.** Most people with sustained hypertension develop LVH as the ventricular muscle thickens in an attempt to force blood beyond the constricted arteriolar beds; thus an S_4 appears when this condition is moderately advanced.

RVH

The least often encountered of the common causes of a fourth heart sound is RVH, but it occurs in a significant number of people, especially those with COPD who develop cor pulmonale. The main pathophysiological feature associated with RVH is **pulmonary hypertension;** thus any disease that produces this condition may result in a right-sided S_4. Right-sided fourth heart sounds can be found to the right of the apex near the lower left sternal border (LLSB).

Ischemic heart disease

The term "ischemic heart disease" refers to the spectrum of coronary artery disease ranging from angina pectoris to myocardial infarction, as well as to other diseases that result in decreased oxygen flow to the heart muscle. Although the mechanism is not completely clear, the area of reduced oxygenation loses some of its compliance, and the more rigid ventricular wall emits an S_4 when blood from atrial contraction strikes it. Thus an S_4 is audible during an acute attack of angina but then fades as the pain subsides; it is also present during the acute phase of an MI until healing of the infarcted area begins to take place. Note that the common denominator in the above conditions is decreased compliance of the ventricular walls.

A knowledge of the fourth sound can be useful in assessment because it has been observed that in many instances improvement of the client's condition is associated with (1) fading of S_4 and (2) decreasing distance of S_4 from S_1. Generally, S_4 becomes louder as the illness worsens, sometimes becoming as loud as

S_1, and diminishes as the client's health improves. In addition, unlike S_3, which always maintains a fixed relationship to the normal heart sounds, S_4 tends to separate farther from S_1 during illness (the interval between the two sounds is relatively spacious) and then moves back toward the first sound as clinical improvement proceeds (approaching the range of a split S_1).

In general, the development of an S_4 is not as serious as the development of an S_3. Since the fourth sound is relatively more sensitive to ventricular stiffening than is S_3, an S_4 appears with lesser grades of ventricular wall firmness. An S_4 does not imply heart failure, as does the appearance of an S_3. In many of the diseases known to be associated with an S_4, the fourth sound may vanish and be replaced by a third sound as the client's condition deteriorates. An example is arterial hypertension, in which an S_4 may be heard for years. As the client's condition worsens, especially with the advent of heart failure, the S_4 may disappear, and in its place an S_3 may be heard. If the failure is successfully treated, the third sound disappears and the fourth sound reemerges. Sometimes an S_3 will appear in a failing heart, and then an S_4 will appear still later for obscure reasons, so that all four heart sounds can be heard. This is fortunately uncommon, for it signals a severely diseased heart.

EXERCISE (*see Appendix E for answers*)

1. Another name for the S_4 is the _____ sound.

2. S_4 occurs late in diastole, immediately before _____.

3. S_4 occurs during _____ of the ventricles as the atria contract and force extra blood into the ventricles.

4. The most common cause of an S_4 is _____.

5. Since S_4 is a sound of _____ pitch, it is best detected by the _____ of the stethoscope.

6. As someone ill with cardiovascular disease improves, S_4 tends to move _____ to S_1.

7. In a client with an MI, an S_4 that grows fainter as time passes probably means that the client's health is _____.

8. An S_4 as an isolated finding is normal in someone over _____ years of age.

9. Like S_3, S_4 is probably the result of decreased ventricular wall _____.

MODULE 23

Gallops

As indicated in the two previous modules, the inclusion of an S_3 or and S_4 in a cardiac cycle gives a triple rhythm that sometimes bears a resemblance to a horse's hoofbeats, particularly at rapid heart rates (Fig. 23-1). It has been the custom since these sounds were first described in the last century to call a third or fourth heart sound a gallop if the heart rate is fast and if indeed the *cadence* of a cantering or galloping horse can be heard. An S_3 or S_4 that indeed *sounds like* a gallop is somehow supposed to be more serious than one that does not possess the clippety-clop of a racing horse. This view has recently undergone considerable criticism for the following reasons:

1. Third and fourth heart sounds do not actually sound very much like the galloping of a horse, unless, of course, the animal one has in mind has only three legs. There is thus inevitable disagreement about when an S_3 or S_4 should be called a gallop. If two observers auscultate a subject at the same time and agree that a third or fourth sound is present, one observer may say that it *sounds* like galloping hoofbeats, and the other may say that it has no gallop cadence at all.

2. It has been found that when an S_3 or S_4 is present, the heart rate makes very little difference in the prognosis or the treatment (unless, of course, the heart rate is so fast that the heart is weak and tachycardiac). The important question is whether or not the S_3 or S_4 is present. Consequently, the trend nowadays is either to call all third and fourth sounds gallops regardless of the heart rate and apparent cadence or else to simply state that an S_3 or S_4 is present. As has recently been said, perhaps the horses ought to be permanently stabled.

If a gallop is heard, it may be easy to identify the extra sound as being in diastole, but it may be more difficult to pin down whether it is a third sound or fourth sound. The problem can be resolved in two ways. First, mentally repeat each of the words "Kentucky" and "Tennessee" several times to see whether one of them seems to match the pattern of sounds being heard. "Kentucky" has a pronunciation pattern similar to an S_3 gallop, whereas "Tennessee" mimics an S_4 gallop. Note that the accented syllable in the names of both states represents S_2, which, as was pointed out earlier, is snappier and of higher pitch than S_1. To get the "feel" of the two rhythms, repeat each of these words several times aloud while comparing them. Second, one can *time* the sounds by palpating the carotid

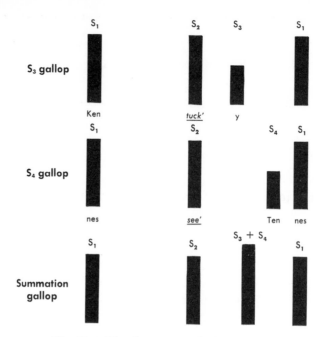

Fig. 23-1. The three types of gallop rhythm.

pulse. S_3 occurs about a third of the way through diastole and S_4 at the end of diastole, almost reaching S_1. S_4 can be heard just before the carotid pulse begins to rise and S_3 just after it has collapsed.

Occasionally, in a severely failing heart, it may happen that both an S_3 and an S_4 will occur together in the same person, giving a quadruple, or cogwheel, rhythm. This gallop is the one that most closely resembles true hoofbeats and can be represented by "tuh-lubb-dupp-uh." Happily, this truer gallop sound is not common. When a combined S_3 and S_4 gallop occurs in a client whose heart rate becomes genuinely tachycardiac (usually because the heart is very weak), the S_3 and S_4 merge, causing a loud extra sound termed a **summation gallop.** It can be distinguished from other triple rhythms by the fact that the extra sound is generally *louder* than S_1 or S_2, whereas with a plain S_3 or S_4 gallop, the extra sound is usually softer than the S_1 or S_2 it accompanies. The summation gallop, because it is conspicuous, is perhaps the triple rhythm identified most frequently.

EXERCISE *(see Appendix E for answers)*

1. A triple rhythm with a cadence similar to the word _____ is an S_3 gallop.

2. S_4 occurs so late in _____ that it is somtimes mistaken for a split _____.

3. When an S_3 and an S_4 merge, the rhythm is then called a _____ gallop.

4. The word "Tennessee" suggests the cadence of an _____ gallop.

5. A summation gallop can be distinguished from simple S_3 and S_4 gallops by the fact that its extra sound is _____ than S_1 and S_2.

MODULE 24

Review one

1. List the four cardinal symptoms of heart disease:

   a. _____

   b. _____

   c. _____

   d. _____

2. State the Cardinal Principle of Chest Pain: _____

   _____

3. Shortness of breath is most often a symptom of _____ .
4. List the five dimensions of pain:

   a. _____

   b. _____

   c. _____

   d. _____

   e. _____

5. Check the statement(s) that reflect(s) inappropriate use of denial:
   A. "I don't care what anybody may say, I know that when my heart attack is fully healed, I'm going back to work!"
   B. "It couldn't have been a heart attack because the pain went away so fast."
   C. "This heart attack hasn't upset me in the least."
6. The two chief ways in which anxiety can distort the history are

   _____ and _____ .

7. Dependent edema is a feature of _____-sided heart failure.

8. The most common cause of peripheral cyanosis is a _____ .

9. The location of the normal PMI is: _____

   _____ .

NOTE: See Appendix E for answers.

10. The most superior technique of physical assessment for detecting enlargement of the heart is _____ .

11. Describe the locations on the chest wall where abnormal precordial movements might be seen or felt in the following conditions:

    a. RVH: _____

    b. LVH: _____

12. Describe the percussion notes that would be expected over the following structures:

    a. Gastric air bubble: _____

    b. Scapula: _____

    c. Pneumothorax: _____

    d. Normal lung tissue: _____

    e. Pleural effusion: _____

    f. Emphysematous lung: _____

13. The most important clue to LVH is the _____ of the apex beat.

14. Never palpate both _____ arteries simultaneously.

15. Identify the following abnormalities of the arterial pulse contour:

    a. As the BP cuff is deflated, the rate of beats is suddenly heard to double: _____

    b. Strong, bounding, jerking pulse that quickly falls away: _____

    c. The inspiratory systolic BP is more than 10 mm Hg lower than the expiratory systolic BP: _____

    d. A weak, slow-to-rise, prolonged pulse that slowly falls away: _____

16. To prevent false _____ when the stethoscope is used to auscultate arteries, the examiner should avoid pressure.

17. The first consideration as to the origin of jugular venous distention is always

    _____ .

18. During inspection of the neck you note a pulsation, and you cannot decide whether the pulse is arterial or venous. You then palpate the left side of the neck while inspecting the right, and you note that the visible pulsation does *not* coincide with the felt pulsation and, furthermore, that the visible pulsation is seen more clearly in expiration. You conclude that it is a _____ pulse.

19. With the client positioned at an angle of 45°, the venous pulse will not normally be seen higher than _____ cm above the clavicle.

20. The following characteristics describe either the arterial or venous pulse. Match the word "arterial" or "venous" to the following:

    a. Double: _____

    b. Up-and-down: _____

   c. Troughs: _____

   d. Elliptical: _____
21. List the major low-frequency sounds:

   a. _____

   b. _____

   c. _____
22. The four principal heart sounds are thought to be caused by sudden accelerations and

   decelerations of the _____ inside the heart.
23. Identify the side of the headpiece that is used to listen for the following types of heart sounds:

   a. High-frequency: _____

   b. Low-frequency: _____

24. The determining event that gives rise to S_1 and S_2 is _____ of the heart valves.

25. List the locations of the classical auscultatory areas:

   a. Mitral: _____

   b. Aortic: _____

   c. Tricuspid: _____

   d. Pulmonic: _____

26. Closure of the _____ valves gives rise to S_1.
27. State the components of the cardiac cycle in the order in which they are auscultated:

   a. _____

   b. _____

   c. _____

   d. _____

28. S_2 is almost always the loudest of the two normal heart sounds at the _____

   _____ area.

29. As the carotid and apical pulsebeats are felt to rise, the _____ heart sound can be heard.

30. An _____ may be the **first and only** sign that the heart muscle is failing.

31. The area in the 3-LICS adjacent to the sternum is known as _____

   _____.

32. Closure of the _____ valves determines when the second heart sound is heard.

33. To avoid stimulation of a possibly hypersensitive carotid sinus body, the examiner should confine palpation of the carotid artery to the _____ half of the vessel.

34. Noises originating from the _____ side of the heart are heard better in inspiration.

35. In the conduction of heart sounds, identify the type of tissue that is:

    a. Most efficient: _____

    b. Least efficient: _____

36. The area of dominance of S_1 is at the _____.

37. The most likely spot to hear splitting of S_1 is in the _____ area.

38. The most powerful of all the heart sound components is _____.

39. The best place to hear splitting of S_2 is usually the _____ area.

40. The most common cause of an abnormally wide split S_1 is _____.

41. Splitting of S_2 is normal in _____.

42. In LBBB, _____ splitting of S_2 is heard.

43. Fixed splitting is due to a delay in the emptying time of the _____ ventricle.

44. To avoid falsely claiming that an S_2 is split in _____ in a child, ensure that he or she is auscultated in an _____ position.

45. The most common cause of a loud P_2 is _____.

46. Loud $A_2 \rightarrow$ _____/_____ disease.

47. An important characteristic of ASD is _____, _____ splitting of S_2.

48. Identify the heart sounds associated with the following terms:

    a. Atrial gallop: _____

    b. Ventricular gallop: _____

    c. Kentucky: _____

    d. Tennessee: _____

    e. Late diastolic filling sound: _____

    f. Early diastolic filling sound: _____

49. Name the single most common cause of the following heart sounds:

    a. S_3: _____

    b. S_4: _____

50. In a summation gallop, the extra sound is usually *(fainter/louder)* than the accompanying normal heart sounds.

51. S_3 and S_4 are accentuated in the _____ position.

52. The area about which one must search carefully for an S_3 or S_4 is the _____ .

53. The third and fourth heart sounds are louder in _____ circulatory states.

54. A right-sided S_4 develops in the RVH of cor pulmonale, just as it can likewise be found in any other condition in which pulmonary _____ is also a prominent pathophysiological feature.

55. Two changes in S_4 that may mean improvement in the client's condition are:

    a. _____

    b. _____

56. The replacement of an S_4 in a hypertensive person with an S_3 may signal

    _____ .

MODULE 25

Friction rub

The friction rub (Fig. 25-1) is a sound heard when the two layers of the pericardial sac begin to rub against each other because of inflammation. The usual reaction of the pericardial cells to the inflammatory process is to exude a serous fluid, but a friction rub may be heard with or without fluid. All that is necessary for the production of the rub is roughening of the two layers. Friction rubs occur in the following conditions:

1. The localized pericarditis that is a frequent complication of myocardial infarction (post-MI pericarditis, most common type)
2. Generalized pericarditis secondary to a variety of infectious and miscellaneous diseases or trauma to the chest

The sound of a friction rub has been described as having a scratchy, grating, or creaky quality that seems close to the ear. It has been compared to the sound produced when fingernails scratch over a piece of sandpaper, a match is struck, new saddle leather creaks during use, or dry snow crunches under someone's step. It can be simulated by placing one hand over an ear and slowly scratching the back of that hand with a finger of the other hand.

The friction rub has gained a reputation for variability. A rub may be composed of one, two, or three components that correspond to the following heart movements (Fig. 25-2):

1. Atrial contraction
2. Ventricular contraction (occurs with apex beat)
3. The rapid-filling phase of the ventricles in early diastole

Any combination of the components may be heard at any given time, and the number of components (as well as their intensity and site of maximum audibility) has been known to change even over a period of minutes. The triphasic friction rub has been identified as the most common in studies utilizing the phonocardiogram, but often the ventricular filling component is so weak that only the two remaining components (atrial and ventricular contraction) are audible. Thus the usual occurrence is a two-component rub having a to-and-fro quality. The monophasic rub is the least common, and when it is present, it is commonly heard with the apex beat, because ventricular contraction, which is the strongest component, is usually responsible for the rub.

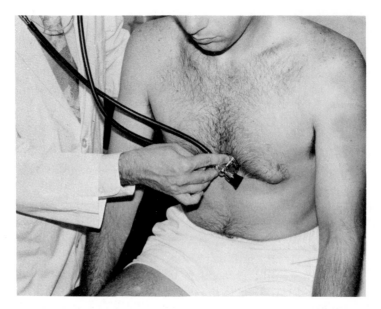

Fig. 25-1. Eliciting the friction rub. If this sound is suspected, it can frequently be brought out by having the client assume the seated flexion position. Since friction rubs tend to be heard best in expiration, it is helpful if the client's breath is held momentarily after exhaling. Explore widely over the precordium, and ensure that the diaphragm of the stethoscope is always in firm contract with the skin. If the diaphragm is applied loosely, respiratory motions of the chest wall may pull the client's skin away from the diaphragm, producing a sound easily mistaken for a rub.

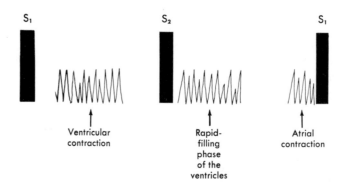

Fig. 25-2. The three components of a friction rub. Each is related to heart movement.

The pericardial rub is frequently a fleeting sound, sometimes being present no more than a few hours, especially after myocardial infarction. Changes in respiration, the position of the client, or pressure applied with the diaphragm of the stethoscope can vary the loudness or quality of the rub. The site where a rub is best heard depends to a considerable extent on the location of the pericardial inflammation; a rub can therefore be heard at various sites such as Erb's point, the lower left sternal border (LLSB), between the LLSB and the apex, and over the xiphoid. Rubs are frequently widely audible over the chest. If the rub is severe, its vibrations can be palpated while the flat of the hand is placed lightly on the chest wall. If faint, it can sometimes be made louder by bringing the pericardium into closer contact with the anterior chest wall; the examiner can accomplish this by having the client lean forward, with the breath held in full expiration, and listening while the diaphragm is pressed firmly into the skin (Fig. 25-1).

It is important to distinguish a *pericardial* friction rub from a *pleural* friction rub, which appears in respiratory conditions such as pleurisy and makes a similar sound. This distinction can easily be made by having the client hold his breath for a few moments; if the rub is of respiratory origin, it will stop at once, but if it is pericardial, it will continue with the cardiac movements. (In a few instances the source of a rub may be *both* the pericardium and the pleurae, at the site where they contact each other, in which case the rub is referred to as pleuropericardial. It is present when the breath is held but is accentuated by respiratory movements.)

The appearance of a friction rub, whether of cardiac or respiratory origin, in a client with myocardial infarction or other heart disease, calls for physician consultation. Clients with MI who are receiving anticoagulants should be watched especially closely for the emergence of a rub. It is possible that the anticoagulants may aggravate the exudation of serous fluid, which may form a pericardial effusion quickly progressing to **cardiac tamponade.** In tamponade the accumulation of fluid surrounds and squeezes the heart so that it cannot contract effectively. Since the amount of fluid that may be fatal is surprisingly small, anticoagulants should be withheld from clients with rubs, pending notification of the physician. Such clients should be observed carefully for the development of tamponade, which may produce the following signs:

1. Rise in JVP (most sensitive indicator)
2. Fall in BP
3. More than 10 mm Hg drop in systolic BP during inspiration (paradoxical pulse)
4. Tachycardia
5. Faint heart sounds
6. Decreased force of the arterial pulses

EXERCISE *(see Appendix E for answers)*

1. A pericardial friction rub can easily be distinguished from a pleural friction rub by having the client _____ momentarily.

2. A friction rub appearing in a client receiving anticoagulants may signal the development of a pericardial _____ .

3. The danger of pericarditis in someone receiving anticoagulants is that the effusion may rapidly progress to _____ .

4. The most sensitive indicator of a beginning tamponade is an elevated _____ .

5. A friction rub can be heard more clearly by having the client lean forward and hold the breath in full _____ .

6. The usual clinical occurrence of a friction rub is a _____-component sound with a _____ quality.

7. Monophasic rubs are produced by _____ contraction that can be heard to occur with the _____ beat.

8. The constriction of the heart produced by tamponade may cause the systolic BP to fall markedly during inspiration, a finding known as _____ pulse.

MODULE 26

Clicks

Clicks are sharp snapping or clicking sounds that occur in systole. Since they are high-frequency sounds, they are best heard with the diaphragm of the stethoscope. They are always pathological, although their gravity varies individually from mild to serious. There are two types: ejection and nonejection.

EJECTION CLICK

Ejection click is also called early systolic click or ejection sound. When one is speaking of the heart, the term "ejection" refers to blood being pumped out of the ventricles into the great arterial vessels (aorta and pulmonary artery). As the name implies, the ejection click is heard at the time of ejection, that is, just after S_1. Early systolic clicks are generally associated with conditions that produce (1) **stenosis** (narrowing) of the involved semilunar valve and (2) **dilation** of the affected great vessel. In the case of the former, the click probably results from a sudden upward bulging (doming) of the thickened, stiff valve leaflets, and in the latter, from vibrations of the dilated vessel wall as blood is ejected into them (Fig. 26-1).

An ejection click may arise from either of the semilunar valves. The pulmonic ejection sound is localized to the pulmonic area, or Erb's point, and is sometimes heard only during expiration (in accordance with the principle that right-sided heart sounds are heard more clearly in expiration). The aortic click is frequently heard clearly at the aortic area, but like so many other sounds produced by the aortic valve, it is carried well to the mitral area (apex), where it is in fact generally heard most clearly.

The ejection click occurs so close to S_1 that it is sometimes mistaken for a split first sound. Recall the following facts:

1. Split first heart sounds are not heard with great frequency.
2. When present, split first heart sounds are confined to a small area near the place where the weaker T_1 component is heard, namely the tricuspid area or LLSB.

Therefore, clear auscultation *at the base or apex* of what at first seems to be a split S_1 in many instances is a tip-off to the presence of a click.

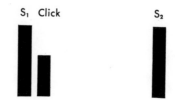

Fig. 26-1. Early systolic (ejection) click.

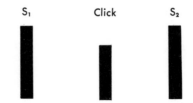

Fig. 26-2. Mid-to-late systolic (nonejection) click.

NONEJECTION CLICK

Nonejection click is also called mid-to-late systolic click. A nonejection click can occur anywhere from halfway to two thirds of the way through systole. The auditory pattern of a nonejection click, together with the two normal heart sounds, can be represented by the lubb-i-dupp sound. A mid-to-late click is usually the result of prolapse of a mitral valve leaflet into the left atrium during ventricular contraction (Fig. 26-2) and can therefore be heard best at the mitral area. The nonejection click is a prominent feature of the **floppy mitral valve syndrome.**

EXERCISE *(see Appendix E for answers)*

1. List the types of click:

   a. _____

   b. _____

2. Clicks are best heard with the _____ of the stethoscope.

3. The mid-to-late systolic click is usually the result of _____ of a mitral valve leaflet into the left atrium.

4. Name the locations where the following sounds are likely to be heard most clearly:

   a. Pulmonic ejection click: _____

   b. Aortic ejection click: _____

   c. Nonejection click: _____

   d. Split S_1: _____

5. Early systolic clicks are associated with:

   a. _____ of the involved semilunar valve

   b. _____ of the affected great vessel

6. Nonejection clicks are an important feature of the floppy _____ syndrome.

MODULE 27

Murmurs

Murmurs are sounds that result from **turbulent blood flow.** Ordinarily, blood flows through the chambers of the heart and the great vessels in straight currents (laminar flow), like water flowing smoothly in a stream (Fig. 27-1). However, if obstacles such as rocks are placed in the path of the flowing stream, the currents are interrupted, producing vortices and giving forth a rushing sound. A similar rushing sound, or murmur, is produced when the laminar flow of the circulating blood is disturbed.

If one attaches a length of surgical rubber tubing about 2 feet long to a laboratory faucet and turns on the water so that a steady stream is flowing through the hose, and then partially pinches the tubing between two fingers, the tubing will begin to vibrate beyond the point of compression because of the turbulence resulting from the water's being forced past the obstacle made by the fingers (Fig. 27-2). In addition, if one simply opens up the faucet gradually, without touching the tubing, the rate of flow increases until a certain point is reached, at which time the flow becomes agitated and the entire length of tubing begins to vibrate. These two situations simulate events that actually occur in the heart and blood vessels in the production of common murmurs.

Examiners who are experienced in measuring blood pressures may have already had occasion to hear a sound resembling a murmur while examining a client with systemic hypertension. As pressure is released on the cuff placed on a person with this condition, it sometimes happens that as blood begins to squirt into the artery under the force of the high blood pressure, a rushing sound can be heard for two or three beats that quickly converts to the usual discrete thumping sounds. Essentially the same phenomenon is at work in a murmur; both the rushing sound and the murmur result from turbulent blood flow.

The sound of a murmur has also been described as a swishing or whooshing noise, and some high-pitched murmurs are said to have a blowing sound. Murmurs are of longer duration than any of the other heart sounds, sometimes lasting throughout the whole of either systole or diastole, and occasionally they can be continuous throughout the entire cardiac cycle. When findings are recorded, "murmur" is abbreviated ⓜ .

Sometimes the vibrations that give rise to murmurs are so great that they are conducted to the chest wall, where they can be palpated with the hand (feels like

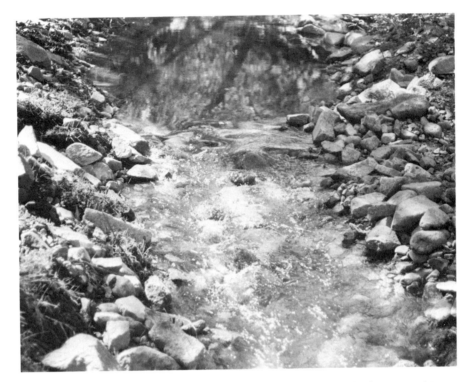

Fig. 27-1. The sound of a murmur has been compared to the sound of water rushing over rocks in a stream.

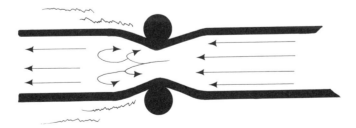

Fig. 27-2. Turbulence produced by crimping a soft rubber hose as water flows through it causes vibration beyond the point of compression.

the purr of a kitten), in which case a **thrill** is said to be present. A thrill can simply be defined as a palpable murmur. Thrills localize the murmurs with which they are associated; that is, the site of the thrill is also the site of maximum audibility of the murmur. When palpating thrills, use a light touch, since too much pressure may block them out. A good technique for palpating thrills and demarcating their extent is to use the fleshy heel of the hand (as in a karate chop). Thrills are produced only as a result of organic lesions and thus are always pathological.

The sources of turbulence that is produced in the flow of blood through the heart and vessels (Fig. 27-3) are as follows:

1. Partial obstruction such as a coarctation (constriction), atherosclerotic plaques, or a stenosed (narrowed) valve opening
2. Increased flow across a normal valve
3. Backward flow through a closed, leaking valve
4. Flow through a hole in the septum between cardiac chambers (provided the hole is not too large)
5. Flow from a vessel into a sharply widened area of that vessel

In the United States the term "murmur" is used to describe turbulent sounds arising from the heart, whereas the term **bruit** (broo'ee) (French word for *noise*) is used for the same kind of sound coming from an artery or organ other than the heart. Bruits can be heard in any artery that becomes narrowed (e.g., carotid arteries with atherosclerotic plaques or arteries affected by renal artery stenosis) or in any tissue that becomes highly vascular (e.g., a vascular tumor or an enlarged, hyperactive thyroid gland). In the United Kingdom the terms "murmur" and "bruit" are frequently used interchangeably to describe turbulent sounds of either intracardiac or extracardiac origin. Murmurs and bruits can be divided into three categories:

1. Systolic
2. Diastolic
3. Continuous (both systolic and diastolic)

Diastolic murmurs are always caused by organic heart disease, and their detection necessitates referral to a cardiologist. Systolic murmurs, on the other hand, may be organic in nature but most often are innocent (benign). Thus timing is crucial in evaluating a murmur. If one is in doubt about which heart sound is S_1 and which is S_2, the methods discussed in Module 14: Cardiac Cycle and Assessment, can be used. Recall that one method of distinguishing the sounds is to notice whether the headpiece of the stethoscope lifts while the murmur is being heard, indicating a systolic murmur. The lift is caused by the rise of the apical beat, which occurs during systole. Continuous murmurs are nearly always caused by organic disease.

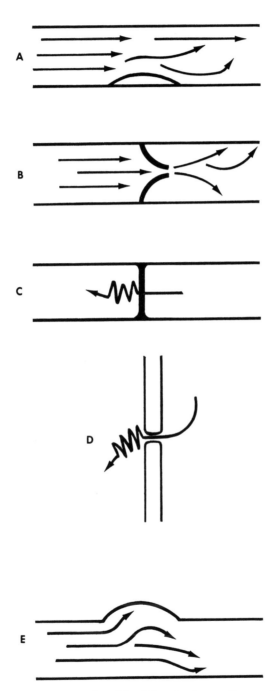

Fig. 27-3. Representations of turbulent blood flow in the cardiovascular system. **A,** Flow past a partial obstruction; **B,** flow through a narrowed (stenosed) valve opening; **C,** backward flow through a closed but leaking valve; **D,** flow through a small hole in a septum; **E,** flow into a sharply enlarged area of a vessel.

EXERCISE (*see Appendix E for answers*)

1. Murmurs and bruits are produced by _____ blood flow.

2. A palpable murmur is called a _____.

3. Check which of the following types of murmurs are almost certainly produced by organic disease:
   A. Systolic without thrill
   B. Systolic with thrill
   C. Diastolic
   D. Continuous

4. Turbulent blood flow is produced by:

   a. Partial _____

   b. _____ flow across a normal valve

   c. _____ flow across a closed, leaking valve

   d. Flow through a _____ in a septum

   e. Flow through a sharply _____ area of a vessel.

5. A murmur heard at the same time the headpiece of the stethoscope lifts upward has to

   be a _____ murmur.

MODULE 28

Describing murmurs

There are seven elements in the description of a murmur: cycle, configuration, location, intensity, quality, radiation, and position.

Cycle

The most important aspect of a murmur is whether it occurs in systole or diastole, since, as has been mentioned, diastolic murmurs are always pathological, whereas many systolic murmurs are entirely innocent. If the murmur occupies only a portion of either systole or diastole, the additional qualifiers "early," "mid," and "late" are used.

Configuration (shape)

The term "configuration" refers to the murmur's level of sound, which assumes a characteristic phonocardiographic pattern according to the amount of turbulence present from moment to moment (Fig. 28-1). Perhaps the easiest configuration to identify is the one created by the *holo*systolic, or *pan*systolic, murmur. This murmur lasts throughout the whole of systole and maintains a level of sound that results in a rectangular diagram (Fig. 28-2). The holosystolic murmur is heard "wall to wall," that is, from S_1 to S_2 without any gaps.

Another commonly recognized shape is the crescendo-decrescendo murmur, which starts with a low level of sound shortly after S_1, quickly builds to a peak at *midsystole,* and then just as quickly fades out, always disappearing before S_2 is reached (Fig. 28-3). This murmur has several other names. Since its peak is in midsystole and there is a gap after S_1 and before S_2, it is called a midsystolic murmur. It is sometimes referred to as a diamond-shaped murmur because of its appearance on the phonocardiogram (Fig. 28-4), and it is also called an ejection murmur, meaning that it is caused by the ejection of blood out of the heart and into the great arterial vessels (Fig. 28-5). A crescendo-decrescendo murmur can be heard in pathological conditions such as aortic stenosis, or it may simply be a result of increased flow across a normal semilunar valve, which would occur in any of the hyperkinetic states (Module 10: Venous Pulse). This latter type of crescendo-decrescendo murmur is called a flow murmur.

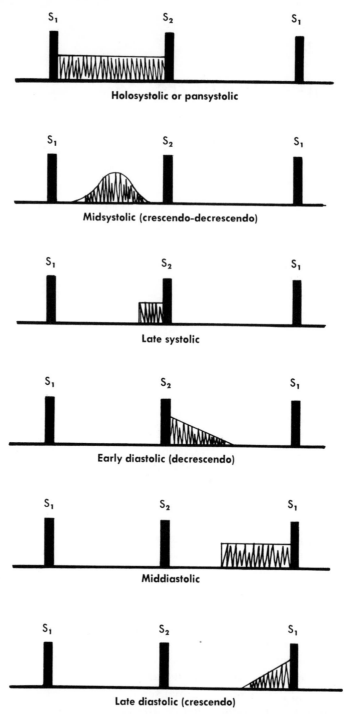

Fig. 28-1. Some common murmur configurations.

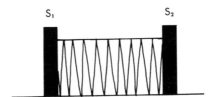

Fig. 28-2. Holosystolic murmur.

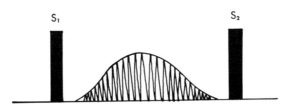

Fig. 28-3. Crescendo-decrescendo (systolic ejection) murmur.

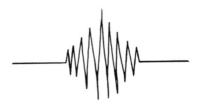

Fig. 28-4. Diamond-shaped appearance of systolic ejection murmur on phonocardiograph.

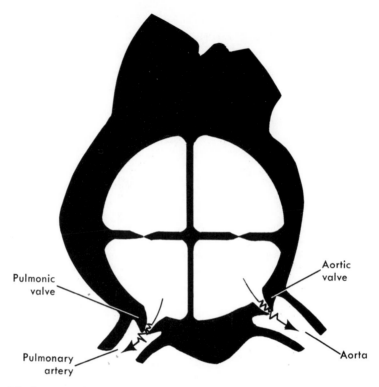

Fig. 28-5. Mechanism of ejection murmur. This type of murmur is heard when one of the semilunar valves is diseased (stenosed) or when there is rapid flow across a normal valve. When the ventricles contract, blood is ejected from the heart into the great arterial vessels. As the ventricles begin to squeeze blood out, the flow across the valve begins to increase (crescendo) until the midpoint of systole, whereupon the flow decreases and the murmur is heard to fade out (decrescendo), disappearing just before S_2.

Location

The point of maximum audibility is referred to as the location of the murmur. It does not necessarily coincide with the source of the murmur. The sounds of murmurs are transmitted in such a way that the site of greatest loudness may be at some distance from the point of origin. Murmurs are transmitted in the direction of blood flow and may be heard louder **downstream** than at the source. For example, some types of murmurs arising at the aortic valve are not heard best in the primary aortic area but rather are loudest on the other side of the sternum at Erb's point (secondary aortic area), along the LLSB or even at the apex.

Intensity (loudness)

Grading the intensity of a murmur is important because in many cases the loudness gives an idea of the severity of the pathology. Many soft systolic murmurs, for example, are completely benign, whereas any murmur intense enough to produce a thrill is certainly the result of organic disease. That intensity correlates with the severity of pathology is only a general rule, however, and one should be aware that there are important exceptions. The murmur of aortic stenosis, for instance, may actually grow softer and even disappear as the condition becomes severe. Septal defects produce murmurs if they are small but may produce no murmur at all if they are large.

Two scales are commonly used for grading the loudness of a murmur. The following six-grade scale is the most widely used in the United States:

Grade 1—very soft; requires a brief period of "tuning in" before it can be heard
Grade 2—soft, but heard right away
Grade 3—moderately loud; no thrill
Grade 4—loud; thrill present
Grade 5—very loud; can be heard when one edge of stethoscope touches chest wall but is not heard if stethoscope is lifted from chest
Grade 6—loudest possible murmur; can be heard even with stethoscope lifted off chest wall

A difficulty with this system is that it contains so many steps that some of them tend to "blend together" because of subjective factors, especially the first two, the second and third, and the last two. There is actually little practical difference between grades 5 and 6, and fortunately the true grade 6 murmur is rare, being found only in drastically ill hearts. Since faint murmurs are so widespread in the population, one commonly sees "grade 1-2 murmur" written in client records (even though these grades are by definition mutually exclusive) when the words "very soft" would describe the murmur just as well.

The simpler and quite satisfactory four-grade scale is popular in the United Kingdom:

Grade 1—very soft
Grade 2—soft
Grade 3—loud; thrill present
Grade 4—very loud

This method is consistent with the grading of all other physical findings that vary along a range; that is, four steps are used. Some authorities recommend using a six-grade scale for systolic murmurs and a four-grade scale for diastolic murmurs. Whichever scale is used, one's observation is recorded as a fraction with the second digit indicating the number of steps in the scale; for example, "grade 3/6" means the third of six grades.

Quality (character)

As Turner (1972) has pointed out, a mere five terms are sufficient to describe the character of the majority of murmurs: blowing, harsh (or rough), rumbling, high-pitched, and low-pitched. Fanciful language is to be avoided in describing murmurs. The more imaginative the description, the more it tends to mislead.

Radiation

Some murmurs are localized to one small area, but others are transmitted to other areas of the chest, to the neck, and even to the back or epigastrium. Whenever a murmur is auscultated, the entire precordium and these other structures must be searched to map out any radiation. Mapping out the pattern of radiation can sometimes be the key to identifying the murmur. For instance, the murmurs of aortic stenosis and mitral regurgitation may both be heard as systolic murmurs that are loudest at the apex. A distinguishing feature in this case is the radiation pattern. In both types of murmurs the radiation is *in the direction of blood flow*, thus the murmur of AS radiates into the carotid arteries, and the murmur of MR is conducted toward the left axilla.

One must bear in mind that radiation frequently is a function of the intensity of the murmur—a very loud one may be heard all over the chest, whereas a soft one may be confined to only one spot.

Position

The position in which the client is placed to elicit the audibility of a murmur is recorded. The following are examples of recording (after reading the modules on the valve lesions, see whether you can identify the murmurs):

1. Grade 2/4 low-pitched, rumbling middiastolic murmur with crescendo accentuation in late diastole, localized to the apex, and heard only when the client is in the left lateral decubitus position
2. Grade 4/6 harsh holosystolic murmur heard loudest at the apex and radiating to the left axilla
3. Grade 1/4 blowing early diastolic murmur best heard at the aortic area, with the client leaning forward and the breath held in full expiration

---

EXERCISE *(see Appendix E for answers)*

1. The most important aspect of a murmur is the part of the cardiac cycle in which it occurs, since _____ murmurs are sometimes innocent, whereas _____ murmurs are always pathological.

2. A holosystolic (pansystolic) murmur has a _____ shape.

3. A midsystolic murmur has a _____ shape.

4. A functional crescendo-decrescendo murmur that occurs in hyperkinetic states is also

   called a _____ murmur.
5. Murmurs are transmitted in the direction of blood flow and therefore may be louder

   _____ than at the source.
6. On the six-grade scale, a murmur that requires a brief period of "tuning in" before it

   can be heard is grade _____.
7. On the six-grade scale, a very loud murmur that ceases to be heard when the stetho-

   scope is lifted off the chest is grade _____.

MODULE 29

Innocent murmurs

The finding of a murmur is not necessarily a cause for concern. In fact, the majority of murmurs one encounters are insignificant systolic murmurs. This is especially true of the very old and very young (Fig. 29-1). Many people, as a normal part of aging, develop some sclerosis on the cusps of the aortic valve, which gives rise to a systolic murmur heard over the primary aortic area (Module 32: Aortic Stenosis and Sclerosis). The majority of children develop a systolic murmur, usually centered about the left sternal edge, at some period during childhood, but the murmur later disappears. Some authorities say that virtually all children develop such innocent murmurs at one time or another in childhood. It

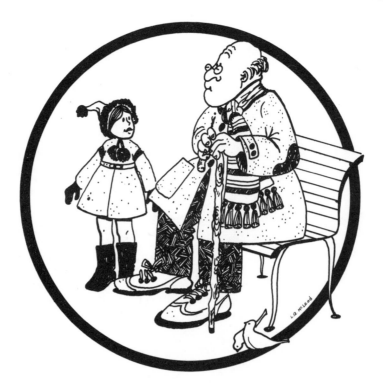

Fig. 29-1. The pediatric and geriatric populations are the two age groups in which innocent murmurs are most commonly found.

is believed that the cause of these murmurs in children is the cramping of the chest contents in their small thoracic containers.

In either adults or children a functional systolic murmur called a flow murmur can be brought about by any hyperkinetic state. Ordinarily the flow of blood over normal semilunar valves does not produce sound, but increased flow across these valves can generate a faint crescendo-decrescendo systolic murmur. The presence of such a murmur is an important assessment feature in patients with fever, anxiety, thyrotoxicosis, or anemia, for if the nursing and medical interventions in these conditions are successful, the murmur can be expected to disappear.

In a person of any age a murmur must have certain characteristics to be considered innocent. It must always occur in systole **(never diastole),** occupy only a portion of systole **(never be holosystolic),** and be soft **(never over grade 2/4 or accompanied by a thrill).** A benign murmur is always accompanied by normal first and second heart sounds. A final requirement is that the murmur must be an *isolated* finding, supported by a negative electrocardiogram and chest x-ray film. In summary, the following are the characteristics of an innocent murmur:

1. Short, soft, systolic ("three S's")
2. S_1 and S_2—both normal
3. ECG and CXR—both normal

EXERCISE *(see Appendix E for answers)*

1. A benign systolic murmur can often be heard in the elderly at the _____ area.
2. An innocent systolic murmur can often be heard in children at the _____ edge.
3. A functional systolic flow murmur can often be brought about by any _____ state.
4. The "three S's" are _____ , _____ , and _____ .
5. To qualify as innocent, a systolic murmur must be an _____ finding.
6. In hyperkinetic states, murmurs are produced when an increased amount of blood flows across the _____ valves during ventricular contraction.
7. Your client, Mr. N. Erviss, has recently had an operation, and his postoperative course has been complicated by an infection. Today you note that he has spiked a high fever and become very anxious, fearing that he is going to die. During auscultation you also note that he has a short, soft systolic murmur that he did not have yesterday. You immediately take measures to reduce his fever and allay his anxiety. It can be inferred that your interventions were successful if the murmur _____ .

MODULE 30

Infectious diseases that produce murmurs

BACTERIAL ENDOCARDITIS

In bacterial endocarditis (BE), wartlike growths of bacteria called vegetations form colonies on the endocardial lining of the heart valves and "chew up" leaflets, causing the valves to disturb the flow of blood, which gives rise to murmurs. Valves with congenital defects or damage from disease such as rheumatic fever are prone to colonization by bacteria. Blood is normally sterile, and if bacteria invade the bloodstream (as they usually do during invasive procedures such as dental extraction or catheterization of the bladder), the body's defenses destroy them in a short time and the blood once again becomes sterile. If there are breaks in the endocardial lining, however, vegetations may begin to form on them. The vegetations are composed of platelets and fibrin that shield the bacteria from the body's defenses and even antibiotics. Once begun, the vegetations continually seed the bloodstream with bacteria, causing fever. Normal valves with intact endothelium are not usually affected, but overwhelming bacterial invasion, which may occur during "mainlining" of addicting drugs with contaminated needles, may colonize even normal valves, especially the tricuspid (Fig. 30-1). The valves most commonly affected in the nonaddict are the mitral and aortic valves.

BE is a serious disease. Before the advent of antibiotics, its diagnosis amounted to a death sentence, and even now the mortality is greater than 25%. The nature of the condition is such that it is often not suspected in persons who have been ill with it for weeks. Early detection is important so that antibiotics can be started before the vegetations have grown so thick that the antibiotics cannot penetrate. Prompt recognition and treatment considerably reduce the risk of death or severe heart damage.

The formula:

Fever + Murmur → Endocarditis

emphasizes that in every person who is encountered with the combination of fever and a murmur, one's first thought should be endocarditis, so that blood for the necessary serial cultures may be drawn and antibiotics started. Although it is true that in a client with this combination the fever may have another cause and

132

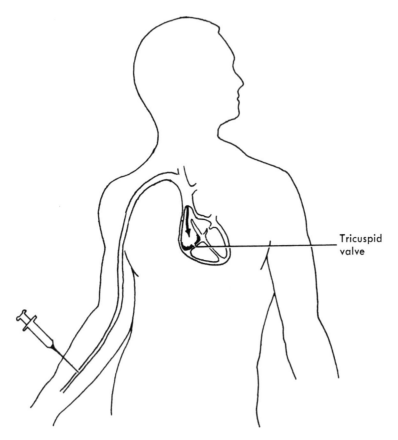

Fig. 30-1. If a drug addict who "mainlines" drugs uses contaminated syringes or needles, the bacterial invasion of the bloodstream may overwhelm and colonize the endocardial lining of a healthy tricuspid valve.

the murmur (if systolic) may simply be a flow murmur caused by the hyperkinetic state of the fever itself, one should nevertheless entertain the suspicion of endocarditis until it is firmly ruled out. **Think endocarditis.**

Murmurs in BE tend to be variable in intensity from day to day, probably because of fluctuations in the fever and anemia that accompany the disease. However, curing the endocarditis results in disappearance of the fever and anemia and even if there is permanent valve damage, there should be some abatement in the murmur as recovery takes place. The day-to-day progress of the murmur needs to be monitored and documented. The development of a *new* murmur or a friction rub is an untoward sign suggesting the advance of active infection.

For prevention of BE, persons with certain types of valvular heart disease are given penicillin or alternate antibiotics just before and after a dental or other minor surgical procedure.

RHEUMATIC FEVER

Rheumatic fever (RF) is another disease that attacks heart valves and causes murmurs. Its victims are usually children from 5 to 15 years of age. RF is essentially an inflammatory reaction to a previous infection with group A beta-hemolytic streptococci; the infection usually takes the form of a sore throat. "Strep throat" is a great deceiver that all is well, because it always goes away whether it is treated or not. If it is not treated with penicillin, however, signs of RF may begin to appear in 2 or 3 weeks, although in some persons the disease may smoulder for years without producing symptoms, and the victim may be well into adulthood before valve damage becomes evident. Of course, the best strategy is prevention of RF by eradicating streptococcal infections, but if acute bouts of RF are intercepted early, valvular damage can be minimized by proper treatment.

The formula:

$$\textbf{Child + Fever + Murmur} \rightarrow \textbf{RF}$$

stresses that in all children who appear with the combination of fever and any murmur, one is obliged to suspect RF. This is true even in the case of soft systolic murmurs, even though we know that this type of murmur can simply be the result of the feverish state of the child, whose very age disposes to such a murmur even when he is healthy. The favorite targets of RF are, first, the mitral valve and, second, the aortic valve.

In the acute episode of RF, assessment is based on the pathophysiological features, which are (in increasing order of severity) endocarditis, myocarditis, and pericarditis.

Endocarditis

Inflammation of the endocardial lining gives rise to the valvular damage and the murmurs. RF is frequently accompanied by anemia, and the fluctuation in the anemia and fever can cause the murmurs to vary. Daily progress of the murmur should be recorded. Since people who have had an attack of RF are susceptible to further attacks with the possibility of more valve damage, they are placed on lifetime prophylactic therapy with penicillin.

Myocarditis

If the myocardium becomes involved, there will be signs of cardiomegaly and CHF.

Pericarditis

Pericarditis is a serious event and is signaled by the development of a friction rub. The social factors in the client's illness should be assessed, since RF tends to be "passed along" from one family member to the next and frequently occurs in a setting of overcrowding, poor sanitation, poor nutrition, and poor access to transportation and health care services.

EXERCISE *(see Appendix E for answers)*

1. Fever + Murmur → _____ .

2. Child + Fever + Murmur → _____ .
3. In BE the wartlike growths of bacteria on the endocardial lining of the heart valves are

   called _____ .
4. For prevention of BE, persons with valvular disease are given penicillin at the time of

   _____ or other minor surgical procedures.
5. RF develops as a response to a previous infection with group A beta-hemolytic

   _____ .

6. Match the signs in column A with the pathophysiological features of RF in column B:

A	B
a. Friction rub	A. Endocarditis
b. S_3	B. Myocarditis
c. Murmur	C. Pericarditis

MODULE 31

Valvular heart disease

Valvular heart disease is either congenital or acquired. If congenital, the most common cause is aortic or pulmonic stenosis or one of the anomalies discussed in Module 42: Cardiovascular Assessment in Children. If acquired, the most likely cause is RF. This was especially true years ago, but now that treatment with penicillin is widely available, valvular disease caused by RF is on the decline. However, in certain areas where the traditional health care system has not penetrated adequately, rheumatic valvular disease is perhaps as common as ever. Another important cause of valvular disease in the past has been syphilis, which has been reported as declining, again thanks to penicillin, but the current epidemic of venereal disease and the increasing problem of bacterial resistance to penicillin may in time result in a resurgence of syphilitic valvular disease. A third important cause is BE, and health care providers who serve populations in the inner cities or other socioeconomically depressed areas should be alert for valvular disease in clients who have a history of "mainlining" drugs. Still other causes are various systemic inflammatory diseases.

When diseases such as those described above attack heart valves, the inflammation results in scarring, and the valves become either **stenotic** or **regurgitant** or both (Fig. 31-1). In stenosis (Greek word meaning *narrowing*), the edges of the valve leaflets become stuck together by the scarring process. The result is a narrowing of the valve opening, which continues to reduce in size with time. In regurgitation the scarring process causes the leaflets to shrink and retract so that they cannot close properly, allowing blood to leak backward (regurgitate) through the valve. Synonyms for regurgitation include insufficiency, incompetence, and reflux.

In the modules that follow, the common valvular lesions and their assessment are described. The lesions described are also prototypes of other lesions not mentioned in this book. For instance, the murmur of tricuspid stenosis is similar to that of mitral stenosis, except that the former is heard on the right side of the heart and the latter on the left.

Although either stenosis or regurgitation is sometimes found alone, the two kinds of lesions often occur together in the same valve. If they are present together, stenosis is usually heard in one half of the cardiac cycle and regurgitation

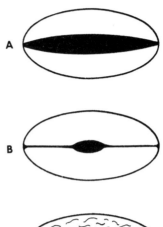

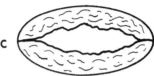

Fig. 31-1. The mitral (bicuspid) valve: **A,** normal; **B,** stenotic; **C,** regurgitant.

in the other half. The result may be a "to and fro" quality in the combined murmurs. In addition, since murmurs are propagated in the direction of blood flow, when stenosis and regurgitation are combined the murmurs of each of these phenomena tend to be heard "in opposite directions." For example, in aortic valve disease in which both phenomena happen to be present, the stenotic murmur tends to radiate forward into the carotid arteries, whereas the regurgitant murmur radiates backward toward the apex.

EXERCISE *(see Appendix E for answers)*

1. Name three infectious diseases often responsible for valvular damage:

   a. _____

   b. _____

   c. _____
2. The scarring process in valvular damage may cause the valves to become either

   _____ or _____ .

3. Since murmurs are propagated in the _____ of blood flow, the murmurs of stenosis and regurgitation originating at the same valve are heard "in opposite directions."
4. The combination of stenotic and regurgitant phenomena at the same valve gives a

   _____ quality to the murmur.

MODULE 32

Aortic stenosis and sclerosis

AORTIC STENOSIS

The aortic valve is normally composed of three half-moon-shaped (semilunar) leaflets. The most common cause of aortic stenosis (AS) is a congenital **bicuspid** valve in which the two leaflets fuse together, reducing the area of the valve opening (Fig. 32-1). This condition may present severe difficulties in infancy or childhood, but more often it produces no problem until the individual reaches middle or old age. Virtually the only other cause is rheumatic fever. The following are the three hallmark symptoms of AS (Module 1: Taking the Heart History: Physical Aspects):

1. Angina
2. Effort syncope
3. Dyspnea on effort (DOE)

The difficulty of the passage of blood through the stenosed valve opening (Fig. 32-2) is responsible for the assessment features: small arterial pulse, narrow pulse pressure, ejection click, soft A_2, delayed A_2, increased and displaced apex beat, and a characteristic murmur.

Small arterial pulse

The upstroke of the carotid pulse is delayed (prolonged) in early AS, and this delayed pulse progresses to **plateau pulse** in late AS (Module 9: Arterial Pulse). In advanced AS the radial pulse may be almost obliterated.

Narrow pulse pressure

A typical BP reading is 105/90. The low systolic BP is caused by the reduced volume of blood being ejected into the periphery. "Runoff" is the term used for the propulsion of blood from the heart through the arteries and its absorption into the capillary and venous beds. In the normal heart, runoff is well into the periphery by the time systole is over, but in AS, blood is still being ejected out of the left ventricle until the very end of systole. Thus, by the time diastole has arrived, runoff has not progressed sufficiently and the blood is still largely in the arteries, accounting for the elevated diastolic BP.

138

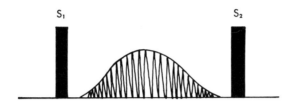

Fig. 32-1. Aortic stenosis produces a midsystolic crescendo-decrescendo murmur.

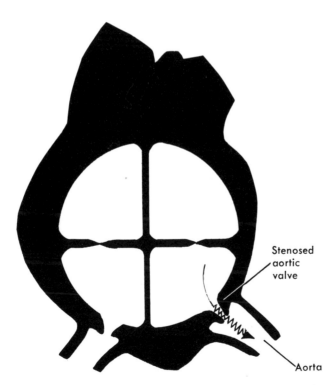

Fig. 32-2. In aortic stenosis, blood is ejected from the left ventricle into the aorta through the narrowed aortic valve during systole.

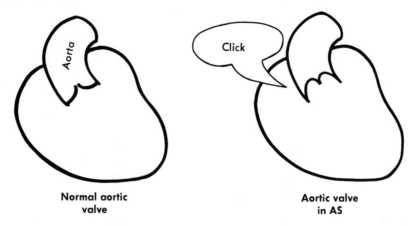

**Normal aortic
valve**

**Aortic valve
in AS**

Fig. 32-3. Mechanism of production of the aortic ejection click in AS. **A,** Position of normal aortic valve leaflets a moment before opening (silent). **B,** The thickened cusps in AS sometimes "dome up" just before opening, producing an early systolic click that is immediately followed by the murmur.

Ejection click

Ejection click (Fig. 32-3) is probably caused by the ballooning up (doming) of the rigid leaflets at ejection (Module 26: Clicks). It may or may not be present, and it disappears as the AS becomes severe.

Soft A$_2$

The aortic component of the second sound is of normal intensity in the early stages but diminishes or disappears with increasing severity of the AS. P$_2$ then becomes relatively louder (recall that P$_2$ > A$_2$ in an adult is always abnormal).

Delayed A$_2$

The soft A$_2$ may become so delayed by prolonged ventricular contraction that **paradoxical splitting** of the second sound may occur (Module 20: Splitting of Second Heart Sound).

Increased and displaced apex beat

To overcome the obstruction to blood flow posed by the stenosed valve, the muscle mass of the left ventricle increases in size (Module 6: Palpation).

Murmur

The following are characteristics of the murmur caused by AS:
1. Midsystolic (crescendo-decrescendo, diamond-shaped, ejection)
2. Harsh (often described as rough or rasping)

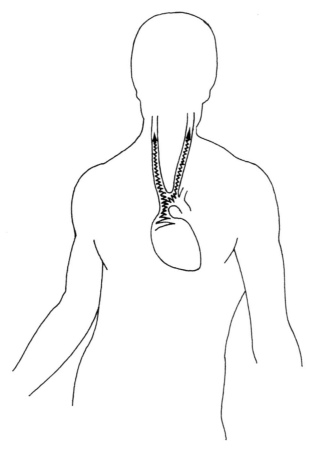

Fig. 32-4. Murmur of aortic stenosis radiates in direction of blood flow into carotid arteries.

3. Usually heard best in the aortic area (occasionally loudest at the apex)
4. Often heard widely over the entire chest
5. Often radiates into the carotid arteries (in the direction of turbulence) (Fig. 32-4)
6. Loudness unrelated to severity
7. Often transmitted well to the mitral area, where it has a more high-pitched, musical quality than at the aortic area (This characteristic has misled some examiners to label the murmur heard in the mitral area as mitral regurgitation. In the case of a systolic murmur heard at the apex, the way to distinguish AS from MR is to recall that AS is diamond shaped and has gaps following S_1 and preceding S_2, whereas MR has a constant sound level that is *pan*systolic, or "wall to wall.")
8. Frequently associated with a thrill over the base of the heart

AORTIC SCLEROSIS

Aortic sclerosis is an insignificant but common condition caused by the process of atherosclerosis in a normal aortic valve of three leaflets. It produces a murmur that is frequently found in elderly persons. The name of this condition is always written out fully to avoid confusion with aortic stenosis, whose abbreviation has been established by convention as AS. Aortic sclerosis has been nicknamed the "50-50" murmur because as many as 50% of persons over the age of 50 years may have one. The murmur resembles that of aortic stenosis, but this benign murmur can be distinguished by four important differences:

1. Soft—does not have the harsh quality of AS
2. Confined to the aortic area
3. No associated carotid pulse abnormalities, as in AS
4. Thrill never present

EXERCISE *(see Appendix E for answers)*

1. The term for propulsion of blood from the heart and its absorption into the peripheral

   vessels is _____ .
2. The three hallmark symptoms of AS are:
   a. Angina

   b. _____

   c. DOE

3. The most common cause of AS is a congenital _____ valve.
4. You are assessing a 65-year-old person who had been identified on a previous examination as having aortic sclerosis. You expect to hear a crescendo-decrescendo murmur at the aortic area, but check which of the following you also expect to find:
   A. Thrill at the base
   B. Soft quality to the murmur
   C. Radiation into the neck
   D. Weak, prolonged carotid pulse
   E. Narrow pulse pressure

5. The characteristic carotid arterial pulse found in late AS is _____ .
6. If A_2 is greatly delayed because of prolonged contraction of the left

   ventricle, _____ splitting may result.

7. The "50-50" murmur is heard in aortic _____ .

MODULE 33

Aortic regurgitation

Aortic regurgitation (AR) is usually acquired and is produced by a variety of infectious, inflammatory, and traumatic conditions.

Rheumatic fever is still perhaps the single most important cause. In AR blood flows backward across the aortic valve; thus the heart must work harder to propel enough blood forward to supply the body's demand for oxygen. As a result, the left ventricle dilates and hypertrophies, but generally the person afflicted with AR does well and seldom has any symptoms until the ventricle goes into failure. Then the signs and symptoms of left-sided CHF appear (Module 37: Congestive Heart Failure).

The other classic assessment features are water-hammer pulse, wide pulse pressure, increased and displaced apex beat, and a characteristic murmur.

Water-hammer pulse

The arterial pulse in AR may be so forceful that the pulsations of the peripheral pulses may be visible during inspection, and the head may be seen to bob with each heartbeat. If the stethoscope diaphragm is placed lightly over the brachial or femoral pulses, sounds simlar to pistol shots may be heard, and if pressure on the diaphragm is increased, to-and-fro bruits may be produced. (See Module 9: Arterial Pulse.)

Wide pulse pressure

A typical BP in AR is 175/40. The elevated systolic BP is due to the increased stroke volume produced by the thickened left ventricle. The low diastolic BP is attributed to fast runoff of blood into the periphery, which is especially quick in AR because of backward flow in diastole, which occurs in addition to the forward runoff (Fig. 33-1). In the normal person, when the ventricles are at rest in diastole, the aortic valve is securely closed and the blood traveling forward in the arteries exerts a diastolic pressure of 60 to 80 mm Hg. In someone with AR, however, some of this pressure "escapes" through the leaky valve, and thus the diastolic BP is kept from building up to its normal level.

Increased and displaced apex beat

This finding is explained by LVH (Module 6: Palpation).

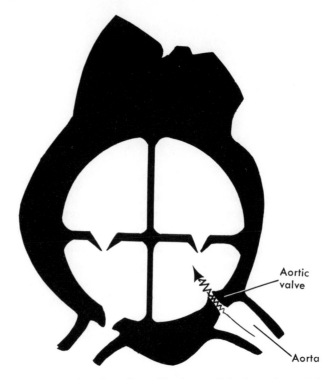

Fig. 33-1. Incompetent aortic valve allows blood to spill backward into left ventricle, generating murmur of aortic regurgitation.

Murmur

The following are characteristics of the murmur of AR (Fig 33-2):

1. Present in early diastole.

2. Decrescendo configuration (loudest immediately after S_1, and then quickly tapers off).

3. High pitched, blowing in quality. This murmur has the highest pitch of all. In some clients this quality may be sharp and is said to sound like the cawing of a seagull, but more often it is softer and is described as a "whiff." To simulate this latter sound, pronounce the word "awe" while breathing in quickly. The best way to detect this high-frequency murmur is to use sufficient pressure with the stethoscope diaphragm to leave a ring on the skin.

4. Often faint. This murmur is known for its difficult audibility. The best way to hear any aortic murmur is to bring the aorta into as close contact as possible with the chest wall by having the client lean forward, with the breath held in full expiration (Fig. 33-3).

5. Often loudest along the LLSB. Since murmurs are transmitted in the di-

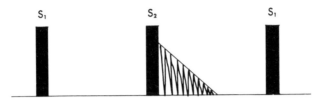

Fig. 33-2. Early diastolic decrescendo murmur of aortic regurgitation.

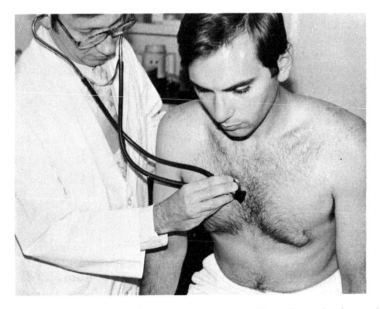

Fig. 33-3. Eliciting the murmur of aortic regurgitation. Client leans far forward to bring aorta into closer contact with precordium and holds breath in full expiration while examiner listens at aortic area and LLSB.

rection of blood flow, the regurgitant jet of blood may conduct the murmur to the sternal edge or even to the apex.

6. Sometimes accompanied by a systolic ejection murmur. This accompanying murmur occurs when there is considerable hypertrophy of the left ventricle. The "muscular" ventricle ejects blood so forcefully across the aortic valve that a crescendo-decrescendo "flow" murmur is created. The combination of the two murmurs has a to-and-fro quality.

Severe aortic regurgitation

If AR becomes severe and CHF sets in, all the signs other than the murmur may be obliterated by the heart failure, and even the murmur may become fainter and shorter. It is more difficult to recognize AR in this situation, but recognition is crucial, since valve replacement is urgently needed.

EXERCISE *(see Appendix E for answers)*

1. Palpable signs of _____ ventricular hypertrophy can frequently be found in AR.

2. The forceful contractions of the ventricle may cause the head to bob with each beat and may produce a systolic _____ murmur at the aortic area in addition to the murmur of AR.

3. AR is generally symptomless until _____ sets in.

4. Describe the runoff in the following conditions:

    a. Aortic stenosis: _____

    b. Aortic regurgitation: _____

    c. Aortic sclerosis: _____

5. The best position for hearing the murmur of AR is
    A. Semirecumbent position
    B. Sitting fully upright
    C. Left lateral decubitus position
    D. Seated flexion position

6. The configuration of the murmur of AR is _____ .

7. The murmur of AR is heard in early _____ by pressing the _____ so firmly into the skin that a ring is left on the skin.

MODULE 34

Mitral stenosis

Rheumatic fever is the only common cause of mitral stenosis (MS). The victim of RF recovers from the acute episode, which may be mild, and there is usually a latent period of 15 to 25 years before the murmur can be detected. The earliest symptoms are hemoptysis and dyspnea (Module 1: Taking the Heart History: Physical Aspects). Since the left atrium must propel blood through a stenosed valve opening (Fig. 34-1), pressure inside the atrium is increased and is then transmitted backward through the pulmonary veins, which tends to congest the capillary beds of the lungs.

The features of assessment are closing snap, opening snap, loud P_2, parasternal lift, and a characteristic murmur.

Closing snap

The term "closing snap" refers to the loud, slapping S_1. Normal, flexible mitral leaflets begin to swing closed in early diastole, but in MS the rigidity of the leaflets holds them open throughout diastole, so that at the last moment in diastole they suddenly and forcefully slam shut. This closing snap can sometimes be palpated in the mitral area. A loud first sound is frequently the first sign of MS. Whenever an increased S_1 is encountered, it should alert one to the possibility of MS.

Opening snap

The opening snap (OS) is a high-pitched, early diastolic sound that is not always present. It is sometimes described as similar to the sound a spinnaker makes when it suddenly fills with air. Opening of the mitral leaflets ordinarily produces no sound, but in MS the stiffness of the cusps abruptly halts their opening movement (almost as if they were tethered), which gives rise to the OS. The OS occurs in diastole because there is always a brief delay after S_2 before the A-V valves begin to open. The OS is nearly always followed by a murmur, and at times the murmur may obscure it. The opening and closing snaps are the hallmarks of MS, and one or both are usually present whether or not a murmur or any other sign is present.

The OS has a tendency to be mislabeled as a third heart sound. As will be recalled from Module 21: Third Heart Sound, this sound, like the OS, is heard at

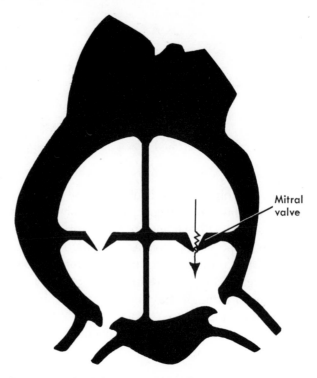

Mitral
valve

Fig. 34-1. Mitral stenosis. Blood flows into the left ventricle during its relaxation phase across a narrowed, rigid mitral valve.

the mitral area and occurs in diastole. Thus one can see how these two sounds are sometimes confused. Although phonocardiographic and other means are sometimes used to differentiate them, the following clinical hints can usually help identify a diastolic sound: timing, pitch, and intensity.

Timing. The S_3 is generally "farther out" in diastole than the OS. The OS occurs 0.08 to 0.12 second after the second heart sound, whereas the S_3 follows S_2 by 0.12 to 0.18 second. As can be seen, there is a slight overlap of the ranges of these two sounds; thus legitimate confusion can indeed take place at times, even in regard to timing.

Pitch. The OS is of high pitch and is well heard with the diaphragm, but the S_3 is a low-frequency sound and as such is often blocked out by the diaphragm.

Intensity. The S_3 is usually a faint thudding sound, whereas the OS is a louder, sharper sound similar to the second heart sound; it does not possess a true "snapping" quality as the name would suggest. Thus, if one hears a diastolic sound that closely resembles the other two sounds, it is probably an OS. The key point in the recognition of a doubtful diastolic sound is that if it is heard well with the **diaphragm** and is **as loud as or louder than** the normal heart sounds, **it almost never can be a third heart sound.**

Loud P₂

Since the blood flowing through the pulmonary artery to the lungs in MS encounters increased resistance in the pulmonary vascular beds, the pressure in the pulmonary artery may be raised (pulmonary hypertension), causing the pulmonic valve leaflets to close forcefully, thus giving rise to the accentuated P_2. At times this closure may be palpable in the pulmonic area of the chest.

Parasternal lift

If pulmonary hypertension is present, the right ventricle may enlarge in an attempt to force blood through the constricted pulmonary vessels (Module 6: Palpation). This may lead to right-sided heart failure (Module 37: Congestive Heart Failure). MS is the only major valve lesion that demonstrates right-sided enlargement. The other three major lesions (AS, AR, MR) display left-sided enlargement (though for three distinctly different reasons).

Murmur

The following characteristics are present in the MS murmur:
1. Long, rumbling, diastolic (**rumbling** quality is the tip-off to MS)
2. Low pitched (as the two other major low-frequency sounds, S_3 and S_4)
   a. Heard best with the bell
   b. Heard at the mitral area
   c. Accentuated in the left lateral decubitus position
   d. Accentuated by hyperkinetic circulation (Thus, mildly exercising the client if there is no acute illness will clarify the murmur; if activity is restricted, having the client cough or squeeze the examiner's fingers will boost the circulation briefly.)
3. Localized to the mitral area (sometimes localized to a small spot, requiring careful search about the apex if MS is suspected)
4. Often accompanied by a diastolic thrill in the mitral area
5. Crescendo accentuated in late diastole (The murmur may become slightly louder just before S_1, as the left atrium contracts and propels an additional amount of blood across the mitral valve. Of course, if the atria do not beat efficiently, as in atrial fibrillation, which frequently accompanies MS, the accentuation is not heard.)

The cadence produced by the combination:

$$S_1 + S_2 + OS + \textcircled{m}$$

can be replicated by repeating "ffoot-ta-ta-rroo" several times. The syllables correspond to the events of MS as shown in Fig. 34-2.

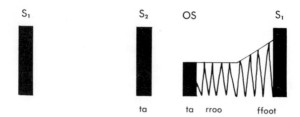

S₁   S₂   OS   S₁

ta   ta   rroo   ffoot

Fig. 34-2. Typical middiastolic murmur of mitral stenosis. Note the late diastolic crescendo accentuation just before S₁. The cadence of this murmur, together with its accompanying heart sounds, is suggested by "ffoot-ta-ta-rroo."

EXERCISE *(see Appendix E for answers)*

1. The hallmarks of MS are

   a. _____

   b. _____

2. The murmur of MS is _____ to the mitral area.

3. If a diastolic sound heard at the mitral area disappears when the diaphragm is pressed firmly into the skin of the chest, it is likely that this sound is *not* a (n) _____.

4. "Closing snap" is a term used for an increased _____.

5. The _____ quality is the tip-off to MS.

6. Name the side of the stethoscope headpiece that is most likely to elicit the following sounds:

   a. Closing snap: _____

   b. Opening snap: _____

   c. Murmur of MS: _____

   d. S₃: _____

7. The cadence of "S₁ + S₂ + OS + ⓜ" is replicated by repeating _____.

8. The murmur of MS can often be clarified by _____ circulation.

9. MS is the only major valve lesion to display enlargement of the _____ side of the heart.

10. There is a tendency to mislabel the OS as the _____.

11. Pulmonary hypertension is associated with the following assessment features in MS:

   a. _____

   b. _____

MODULE 35

Mitral regurgitation

In MR, blood leaks backward through the mitral valve into the left atrium during ventricular contraction (Fig. 35-1). To compensate, the left ventricle hypertrophies so as to be able to propel more blood in a forward direction with each heartbeat and thus satisfy the body's oxygen demand. Although this disease also is commonly termed "mitral insufficiency" or "mitral incompetence," a problem arises in abbreviation, since MI is also the standard abbreviation for myocardial infarction. Thus, to avoid confusion, I prefer to use the term "mitral regurgitation" and its abbreviation, MR.

The usual causes of MR are

1. Rheumatic fever
2. Bacterial endocarditis
3. Papillary muscle dysfunction (Module 41: Myocardial Infarction)
4. Failure of the left ventricle

The latter is the most common cause. When left ventricular failure becomes advanced, the chamber enlarges and dilates to such an extent that the mitral valve ring is stretched open, pulling the leaflets apart and allowing blood to jet backward into the atrium. MR secondary to CHF, which is termed **functional** mitral regurgitation, generally disappears when the heart failure is brought under control.

Except for palpitations, which tend to be a recurrent problem in some individuals with MR, there are usually no symptoms until late in the disease, when CHF supervenes.

The assessment features in MR are soft S_1, increased and displaced apex beat, presence of an S_3, and a characteristic murmur.

Soft S_1

The first heart sound is chiefly produced by the closure of the mitral valve cusps. Since they cannot come fully together in MR, the S_1 is weak or even absent.

Increased and displaced apex beat

The apex beat increases and is displaced because of the hypertrophy of the left ventricle. The findings here are the same as in left-sided enlargement from any other cause (Module 6: Palpation).

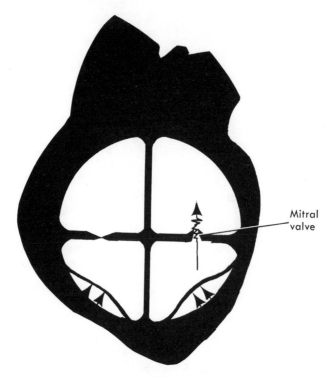

Mitral valve

Fig. 35-1. Mitral regurgitation. During ventricular contraction, blood regurgitates into left atrium through incompetent mitral valve.

Presence of an S₃

A third heart sound may be present, especially if CHF has begun. Even though an S_3 may be normal in someone under the age of 30 years, when it is found in MR it should always be regarded as an unfavorable sign that generally indicates the more severe degrees of MR and possibly decompensation of the left ventricle.

Murmur

The murmur of mitral regurgitation has the following characteristics:
1. Holosystolic (Fig. 35-2)
2. Loudest at the mitral area
3. Radiates to the left axilla (in the direction of the regurgitant jet of blood; see Fig. 35-3)
4. Usually blowing in quality
5. Usually loud (grade 3/4 or louder)
6. Systolic thrill usually present at the mitral area
7. Often spills over onto S_2 and obscures it

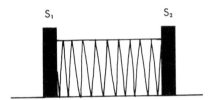

Fig. 35-2. Mitral regurgitation produces a holosystolic (pansystolic) murmur.

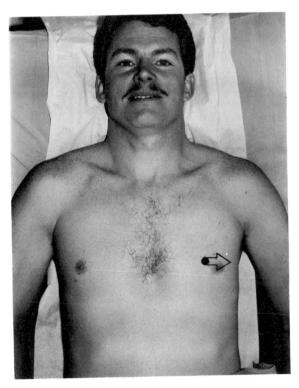

Fig. 35-3. Murmur of mitral regurgitation radiates in direction of blood flow toward left axilla.

EXERCISE *(see Appendix E for answers)*

1. In failure of the _____ ventricle, the hypertrophy and dilatation stretch the mitral valve ring open. This condition is termed _____ mitral regurgitation.

2. In MR the valve leaflets cannot close properly, and therefore the _____ heart sound is decreased.

3. The more severe degrees of left ventricular hypertrophy and dilatation in MR are responsible for appearance of the _____ heart sound.

4. The holosystolic murmur of MR radiates in the direction of the regurgitant jet of blood toward the left _____ .

5. The murmur of MR often spills over onto the _____ heart sound, making it difficult to hear.

MODULE 36

Floppy mitral valve syndrome

Floppy mitral valve syndrome was practically unknown 25 years ago, but it has become the most frequently diagnosed valvular lesion. It is associated with redundancy of one or both mitral leaflets, and it is thought that a degenerative process of unclear etiology may be involved. It is found most commonly in young women.

In this syndrome the mitral valve is competent in early systole, but in the mid or late portion of systole, the redundant leaflet prolapses into the left atrium, giving rise to a sharp, high-pitched click (Fig. 36-1). This nonejection (mid-to-late) systolic click is the hallmark of the condition, which is sometimes called the "mitral valve prolapse–click syndrome." Another term commonly heard is "billowing mitral leaflet syndrome." The click is heard best with the diaphragm of the stethoscope at the mitral area, and together with S_1 and S_2, it sounds like "lubb-i-dupp." Sometimes a murmur of mitral regurgitation can be heard immediately after the click (Fig. 36-2), but this murmur is not an essential feature of the syndrome.

The floppy valve syndrome is often symptomless and is generally benign. No treatment is usually needed; however, antibiotic prophylaxis for BE is administered before dental and surgical procedures and catheterization of the bladder, since it is believed that the affected leaflets are susceptible to colonization by bacteria. It is for this reason that detection is important.

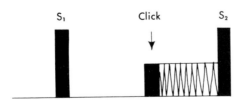

Fig. 36-1. Floppy mitral valve syndrome is characterized by a mid-to-late (nonejection) click that is sometimes followed by a murmur of mitral regurgitation.

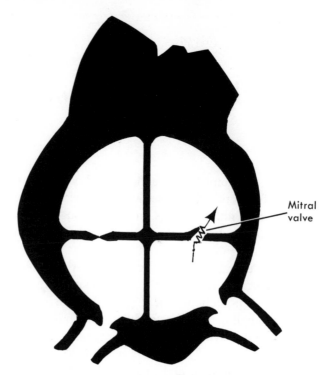

Fig. 36-2. Floppy mitral valve syndrome. In this condition, one of the mitral valve leaflets prolapses into left atrium during latter part of ventricular contraction. This allows blood to leak backward and gives rise to the murmur of mitral regurgitation.

EXERCISE *(see Appendix E for answers)*

1. In floppy mitral valve syndrome, the redundant leaflet _____ into the left atrium during systole.

2. The hallmark of this syndrome is a _____ systolic click.

3. The click is best heard with the _____ of the stethoscope at the _____ area.

4. A murmur of _____ sometimes can be heard immediately after the click.

5. Detection of a floppy mitral valve is important for the provision of antibiotic prophylaxis against _____.

MODULE 37

Congestive heart failure

There are four keys to understanding all the points of assessment in congestive heart failure (CHF), and they are the chief pathophysiological features of the condition:

1. Reduced forward output
2. Myocardial decompensation
3. Enlargement
4. Increased pressure rearward*

CHF is the final common pathway for almost all types of heart disease, including all those discussed in previous modules, and is therefore an important condition. The term "congestion" in CHF is synonymous with "edema." Edema is the hallmark of CHF, and fluid eventually begins to collect in one or another part of the body in this condition. Since the weakened heart cannot pump blood adequately, the blood that is not ejected dams backward through the heart. The result is waterlogging and swelling of the organs that are found rearward from the involved ventricle(s). Fluid accumulation may become extensive before it makes an appearance in the skin. The fact that the body can hold *up to 15 pounds* of fluid before it begins to show accounts for the most important principle of assessment in CHF: **Weigh the client daily.**

To grasp the basis for assessment in this condition, think of the heart as being made up of two separate pumps—the right and left sides of the heart—and divide CHF into left-sided failure and right-sided failure. Although it is unusual to have a CHF that is entirely localized to one side of the heart, it is nevertheless true that most cases are predominantly on one side or the other. The most common type of CHF is left-sided because the left ventricle is usually the first chamber to fail. In fact, the most common cause of right-sided heart failure is a left-sided failure that spills over to the right side (the reverse seldom occurs).

Edema always occurs rearward from the failing ventricle in response to the increased pressure, which drives fluid out into the tissues. Thus one can anticipate which organs will become engorged with fluid by tracing the two pathways of pressure backup (Fig. 37-1), which are summarized as follows:

Left ventricle → *Pulmonary* veins
Right ventricle → *Systemic* veins

---

*In this sense means opposite to the direction of normal blood flow.

158

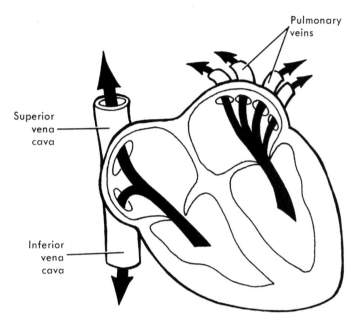

Fig. 37-1. Pathways of pressure elevation in CHF. Congestion of organs can be predicted by tracing pathways. In left-sided failure, pressure backs up through pulmonary veins into lungs, resulting in pulmonary edema. In right-sided CHF, pressure is transmitted upward into superior vena cava, distending neck veins, and downward into inferior vena cava, congesting liver.

Note that all the signs and symptoms in CHF are related to the pathophysiological features.

LEFT-SIDED FAILURE
Reduced forward output

Disorientation. The decreased blood flow to the brain results in cerebral hypoxia, which may bring about an acute confusional state manifested by incoherent speech and **restlessness.** The treatment for this state is not psychotherapy and, above all, not tranquilizers. What the client in this condition needs can be recalled by the mnemonic, "In heart failure, odd behavior calls for ODD medicine—Oxygen, Diuretics, Digitalis."

Nocturia. The kidneys respond to the decreased renal blood flow by conserving sodium, which in turn retains water in the circulation. Initially, this retention can be viewed as beneficial for the heart, since the increased blood volume stretches the heart muscle, which, according to Starling's law, makes the heart beat more effectively. This law, in effect, states that the myocardium has the property of contracting more forcefully as it is stretched, and it holds true up to a point. At that point the Starling effect can simply no longer operate, and then a vicious cycle, diagrammed below, begins:

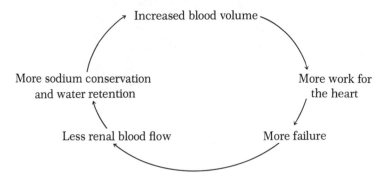

When the Starling effect can no longer compensate for the increased fluid retention, edema begins to congest the tissues of the body. In the early stages of CHF the deposition of fluid in the tissues is more operative during the day, when the client is active. During sleep at night, however, the demands on the heart are less, and the left ventricle is able to pump enough blood to return flow through the kidneys to normal. A diuresis begins that fills the bladder and awakens the client. This sequence of events may occur several times during the course of a night. Once again, the simple question, "How well do you sleep?" may be instrumental in detecting early heart disease.

Peripheral cyanosis. Reduced cardiac output results in sluggish circulation in the periphery. The amount of time the blood stays in contact with any given tissue is thus prolonged, and that tissue is able to extract more oxygen from the blood. By the time the blood reaches the tips of the fingers, toes, nose, and ears, it is fairly well stripped of oxygen and therefore appears blue. Cyanosis in a person with CHF who has been properly warmed is always serious. (See Module 3: Some Important Physical Signs in Heart Disease.)

Cheyne-Stokes respirations. Cheyne-Stokes respirations most often occur in elderly persons and may be the first reason a client with CHF seeks health care. They are frequently first noticed by the spouse, who observes that the client has stopped breathing during sleep. The client may only be aware of nightmares or may simply be conscious that he or she awakens several times during the course of the night or has difficulty sleeping, without being able to specify the exact nature of the sleep disturbance. Again, the question, "How well do you sleep?" may give telling information about the heart. Because of the reduced cardiac output, the respiratory centers of the brain stem are not perfused well with oxygen during sleep, and the characteristic cycle of apnea followed by hyperpnea begins to take place. If barbiturates are prescribed for the client's complaint of not sleeping well and the CHF is missed, the respiratory centers in the brain will be further depressed, aggravating the Cheyne-Stokes respirations.

Myocardial decompensation

Third heart sound. The appearance of S_3 signals increasing tension on the ventricular wall from decompensation of the myocardium. It bears repeating that this sound may be the first and only sign of CHF. If fact, there may be no clue, between the appearance of the third heart sound and the onset of frank pulmonary edema, that CHF is present. Therefore the detection of an S_3 is an especially significant intervention.

Enlargement

Apex beat changes. Enlargement of the ventricle causes (1) an increase in size, force, and duration of the apex beat and (2) a shifting outward and downward (heaves to the left).

Murmur of MR. In advanced CHF the dilatation of the ventricle may cause the mitral valve cusps to separate so that they cannot close fully. When the ventricle contracts, blood flows in a backward direction across the valve into the atrium, producing a holosystolic murmur. This type of MR is not due to an organic lesion of the valve and thus is termed functional mitral regurgitation. If therapy for CHF is successful, the valve ring returns to normal size, the valve is once again competent (closes securely), and the murmur disappears.

Alternating pulse. An alternating pulse consists of a weak arterial pulsebeat alternating with a stronger beat (Module 9: Arterial Pulse). This phenomenon is once again explained by the Starling effect. Since the failing ventricle cannot completely eject the usual amount of blood during the first (weak) beat, it leaves a residual volume that exerts stretch on the ventricular wall and enhances its contractility. Thus the second beat is stronger and empties the ventricle more completely. This sign is specific for an enlarged, gravely ill left ventricle.

Increased pressure rearward

Since the pathway of increasing backward pressure for the failing left ventricle is through the **pulmonary** veins, it is the lungs that become edematous in left-sided failure.

Dyspnea. Evaluate the type and severity of dyspnea. (See Module 1: Taking the Heart History: Physical Aspects.)

Cough. Cough is due to congestion of the bronchioles. It is an early subtle sign of CHF.

Wheezes. High-pitched, musical sounds called wheezes can be heard with the diaphragm of the stethoscope ranging widely over the lung fields on both the anterior and posterior chest. The bronchioles react to the presence of the excess moisture by constricting, and it is the passage of air through the narrowed tube that produces the wheeze. The wheezes usually occur during expiration but may also be heard during inspiration. When they are very marked, wheezes have been described as sounding like "violins screeching." Their occurrence as a result of

CHF proves the adage, **All that wheezes is not asthma.** Think of a cardiac origin first in the client who begins to wheeze for the first time after the age of 50 years.

Pink-tinged sputum. The rupture of fine bronchiolar capillaries results in pink-tinged sputum.

Crackles. Another type of sound detected by auscultation over the lung zones (Fig. 37-2) is called crackles. Other names are crepitations and rales. Normally when the lungs are auscultated, only the sound of the air rushing in and out of the lungs is heard, a sound sometimes described as "a soft breeze rustling back and forth through the trees." In left-sided failure, pressure builds up in the capillary beds of the lungs, forcing fluid to ooze into the normally dry alveoli. This abnormal moisture gives rise to crackling sounds, which are superimposed on the normal breezy breath sounds. The sound of a single crackle can be simulated by wetting the thumb and forefinger and pressing them tightly together. Hold these two fingers close to the ear and then separate them rapidly. A slight snapping sound will be produced. A similar condition occurs in the individual alveolus in left ventricular failure. The walls of the alveoli are moist because of pulmonary edema and stick together when they are relaxed in expiration. When the client breathes in, the inrush of air separates the alveolar walls, creating a snapping sound. The sound of many moist alveoli opening up on inspiration produces a crackling noise that is similar to the sound produced when a piece of cellophane is crushed in the fist. The sound of crackles can also be simulated by pulling down a few strands of hair over the opening of one ear and slowly rubbing them together between two fingers (Fig. 37-3).

Pulmonary edema is a type of dependent edema, and crackles, if present, will therefore be heard in the dependent areas of the lungs. If the client is sitting, they will be heard at the lung bases. If the client is lying on his left side, they will be heard over the left lung, and if on the right side, over the right lung. It is emphasized that crackles are a late sign of CHF, sometimes occurring long after an S_3 or the other early signs and symptoms have appeared. The presence of crackles is generally a serious sign and becomes increasingly serious as the crackles can be heard higher in the lung fields. Likewise, a decrease in the level over the back where crackles can be heard represents improvement.

Dullness at the lung bases. The backup of fluid into the lungs in CHF may appear as pulmonary edema or pleural effusion or both. In both types of abnormal fluid accumulation, gravity causes the fluid to pool in the lung bases, decreasing or even obliterating the normal breath sounds that would be expected there. Pay particular attention to asymmetrical breath sounds, since fluid collection is frequently unequal on both sides. The normal resonant percussion note over the lung bases becomes dull if fluid is present.

Central cyanosis. The accumulation of fluid in the alveolar beds in severe CHF ultimately impairs gas exchange to such a degree that even the tongue and the mucous membranes inside the cheek become bluish. Central cyanosis is an urgent sign in the person with CHF.

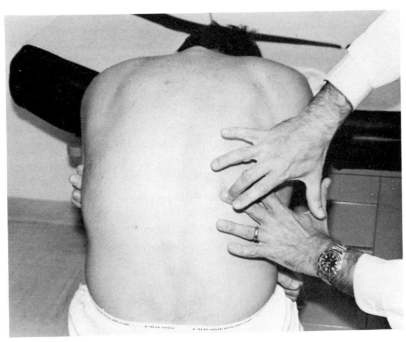

Fig. 37-2. Best position for auscultation of lungs is with client's head and shoulders bowed forward, just as in percussion.

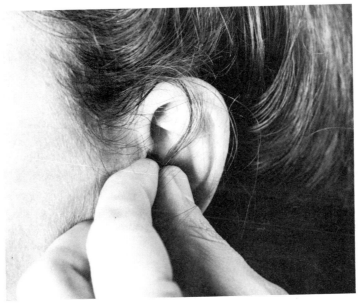

Fig. 37-3. Sound of crackles can be simulated by bringing down a few strands of hair in front of meatus of ear and rubbing them slowly back and forth between thumb and fore-finger.

RIGHT-SIDED FAILURE
Reduced forward output

Hepatojugular reflux. The term "hepatojugular reflux" is a misnomer. This test to assess early right-sided failure would more appropriately be called abdominojugular reflux. It does not form part of a routine physical examination and should be used only when CHF is suspected. Place the client at a 45° angle. Press firmly but gently on the client's upper abdomen. It is not necessary to press directly over the liver, as the name of this test implies. Holding the pressure for 30 to 60 seconds squeezes blood out of the abdominal organs and increases venous return to the right side of the heart. Ordinarily, upper abdominal pressure will distend the jugular veins for a few seconds, but if the right heart is pumping healthily, this distention rapidly disappears. If the right heart cannot pump out its normal volume because of failure, the increased venous pressure will overload it, and the jugular veins will remain visibly engorged during the entire time of compression.

CAUTION: Make sure the client is breathing normally. If the client holds the breath, as many persons do in response to abdominal compression, a false positive result will be obtained.

Myocardial decompensation

Right-sided S_3. When the right ventricle enlarges, a third heart sound may arise from the right ventricle. This sound is the same as a left-sided S_3 except that it is heard more to the right of the apex, near the sternum.

Enlargement

Parasternal lift. A directly anterior movement of the chest wall located just lateral to the LLSB can be seen or felt if there is hypertrophy of the right ventricle (Module 6: Palpation).

Murmur of tricuspid regurgitation. Marked enlargement of the right ventricle may dilate the tricuspid valve ring so that the leaflets cannot close properly. The result is a functional regurgitant murmur similar to that produced by the mitral valve in cases of advanced left-sided failure. The holosystolic murmur of tricuspid regurgitation (TR) sounds very much like that of MR except that it is loudest in the tricuspid area and tends to become louder during inspiration (as do all murmurs that originate in the right side of the heart). TR can also produce abnormal systolic pulsations in the venous system.

When the tricuspid valve is competent, it acts like a closed gate to block the wave produced by ventricular contraction from passing through the venous system. When the valve is incompetent, however, the gate is open and a systolic pulsation travels down the venous circulation. This pulsation is most readily detected at the jugular vein, where it can be seen as a large V wave (Module 10: Venous Pulse). Systolic pulsations of the liver can also be palpated by placing the fingers in the intercostal spaces over the hepatic area, and in some individuals the eyeballs can be seen to pulsate during systole. Once the right-sided failure is corrected, the murmur and venous pulsations of TR will often disappear.

Increased pressure rearward

Jugular venous distention. The internal jugular vein, because of its proximity to the chambers of the right heart, is usually the first site to reflect the elevated pressure of right ventricular failure (Module 10: Venous Pulse).

Liver enlargement. The organ closest to the right heart in the systemic venous pathway is the liver. Thus a swollen, edematous liver is a common finding in right-sided failure. The liver becomes tender, and blunt percussion with the fleshy part of the fist over the hepatic area of the rib cage or touching the edge of the liver under the rib margin causes a painful response. Percussion with the fingertips can usually be tolerated, however, and the area of dull percussion notes will exceed 12 cm in the MCL.

Nausea and vomiting. The stretching of the liver capsule when this organ enlarges causes stimuli to be sent up the vagus nerve to the vomiting center in the brain stem. The very earliest symptom of right-sided failure thus may be the complaint of indigestion. Inducing clients who have failure of the right ventricle to take sufficient nourishment can be a challenging problem.

Ascites. The increased pressure in the portal circulation forces fluid out into the abdominal cavity. The degree of ascites is assessed by daily measurements of the abdominal girth with a tape measure.

Dependent edema. Dependent edema is produced in right heart failure as the pressure in the systemic veins continues to rise, causing fluid to collect in the subcutaneous tissues (Module 3: Some Important Physical Signs in Heart Disease).

EXERCISE (*see Appendix E for answers*)

1. The keys to understanding assessment in CHF are the following four chief pathophysiological features:

   a. Reduced forward _____

   b. Myocardial _____

   c. _____

   d. Increased pressure _____

2. The hallmark of CHF is _____ .

3. State the most important principle of assessment in CHF: _____ .

4. The pathways of pressure backup in CHF are

   a. Left ventricle → _____ veins

   b. Right ventricle → _____ veins

5. Starling's law states that the heart muscle contracts more forcefully when its fibers are _____ .

6. Left-sided failure may dilate the mitral valve ring and produce a functional pansystolic murmur of mitral _____ .

7. High-pitched, musical sounds in the lungs caused by constriction of the bronchioles are called _____ .

8. The sounds of moist alveoli opening up on inspiration are called _____ .

9. If one uses the hepatojugular reflux test to assess early right-sided failure, one must ensure that the client is _____ normally.

10. TR can produce abnormal _____ pulsations in the venous system.

11. The most common cause of right-sided failure is _____ .

12. The auscultatory sign that appears when one of the ventricles begins to decompensate is a(n) _____ .

13. Mr. Wright has suffered from chronic left ventricular CHF for years and is admitted to the hospital for an acute exacerbation. It would be important to watch for crossover of failure to the right ventricle. Check which signs would indicate that crossover might be occuring:

    A. Heaving apex beat

    B. Pretibial edema

    C. Alternating pulse

    D. Jugular venous distention

    E. Increased liver dullness

MODULE 38

Aortic aneurysm

An aneurysm is a weakened area of an arterial wall that "balloons out" (Fig. 38-1). Assessment features are abnormal pulsations, loud A_2, ejection click, vascular compression signs, bruit, and tracheal tug.

Abnormal pulsations

Most abnormal pulsations are often seen in the second and third right intercostal spaces if the aneurysm is in the ascending aorta. If the aneurysm is located at the arch of the aorta, a pulsation may be visible in the suprasternal notch (but this type of pulsation is also found in a kinked carotid artery, a condition that is not uncommon in elderly persons). Check the epigastric area for unusually large pulsations of aneurysms of the abdominal aorta. Follow the midline of the abdomen to well below the umbilicus, first palpating deeply but gently (to avoid rupture of a possible aneurysm) and then auscultating with the stethoscope diaphragm. An aneurysm may be felt as an **expansile mass** over which a systolic bruit may be heard. (NOTE: Some individuals, especially thin persons, have a small pulsation from a normal aorta that can be palpated in the epigastrium.)

Loud A_2

The quality of the loud A_2 has been described as ringing or tympanitic in aneurysms of the ascending aorta.

Ejection click

If there is dilatation of the root of the aorta because of an aneurysm in the ascending aorta, an ejection click may be heard at the aortic area.

Vascular compression signs

If the bulge of the aneurysm compresses the vena cava or innominate vein, there will be unilateral or bilateral engorgement of the neck veins (Module 10: Venous Pulse). If the bulge impinges on adjacent arteries, the pulse to one or both of the carotid arteries may be decreased or delayed. Similar decreases or delays may also be noted in one or both arm pulses (brachial and radial).

167

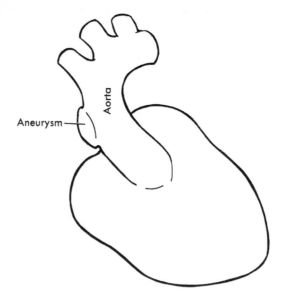

Fig. 38-1. Aortic aneurysm. A saccular type on ascending portion of aorta is depicted here. Out-pouching of vessel wall creates turbulent blood flow, giving rise to a bruit.

Bruit

There is often a loud, harsh systolic bruit best heard in the 2-RICS or 3-RICS. The bruit is usually accompanied by a thrill.

Tracheal tug

Each systolic pulsation of the aneurysm may compress a bronchus in a downward direction. This downward tug can be felt in the trachea by placing a fingertip in the suprasternal notch.

Brief mention must be made of the uncommon but not rare **dissecting aortic aneurysm,** in which a column of blood splits and spreads through the medial layer of the aortic wall. Although an aortic dissection may produce abnormal pulsations and vascular compression signs as described above, it often may be suspected on the basis of the history alone. Sudden, excruciating chest pain is usual. At times the pain cannot be distinguished from that of an acute MI, but at other times there is a characteristic pain history that may include any of the following descriptions of pain:

1. Tearing quality
2. Wide radiation to back and abdomen
3. Changes in location, generally from the center of the chest outward

EXERCISE *(see Appendix E for answers)*

1. If an aneurysm occurs in the ascending portion of the aorta, then a pulsation, a loud A_2, an ejection click, and a bruit are likely to be found in the second _____ intercostal space, also known as the _____ area.

2. If an aneurysm is located at the _____ of the aorta, a pulsation may be seen or felt in the suprasternal notch.

3. The chief vascular compression signs produced by an aneurysm are a decreased or delayed _____ pulse and distention of the _____ pulse.

4. Characteristic pain of a dissecting aortic aneurysm has a _____ quality.

5. An aneurysm of the abdominal aorta may be felt as an _____ near the midline of the abdomen.

MODULE 39

Systemic hypertension

PHYSICAL ASSESSMENT

In addition to the use of the sphygmomanometer, the following points of physical assessment are useful in evaluating the severity of high arterial blood pressure: increased A_2, signs of LVH, and the presence of an S_4.

Increased A_2

The increased arterial pressure causes the aortic valve leaflets to snap back with unusual force; thus the aortic component of the second sound is louder than normal. Because hypertension is such a widespread disease, the possibility of its presence should be entertained as soon as a loud second sound is heard (regardless of location) if a blood pressure determination has not been made prior to auscultation. Once a loud S_2 has been heard, the examiner should then establish which of the two components (A_2 or P_2) is responsible for the loudness of the second sound. This can be accomplished by moving the stethoscope to the pulmonic area, where both components can usually be heard during normal inspiratory splitting. Generally, the higher the BP, the louder the A_2. With successful treatment the A_2 returns to normal intensity.

Signs of LVH

Hypertrophy occurs because the left ventricle must work harder to force blood past the constricted arterioles. Three fourths of all hypertensive persons develop some form of cardiac hypertrophy, which may not go away even if the blood pressure is brought under control. The signs of LVH that can be determined by inspection and palpation are discussed in Module 6: Palpation.

Presence of an S_4

The presence of a fourth sound signals moderate-to-severe hypertension. The single most common cause of a pathological S_4 is hypertension. The S_4 is an early sign of LVH and is usually detected before the palpable signs of ventricular enlargement. When the blood pressure is returned to normal, the strain is taken off the left ventricle, and the S_4 usually disappears.

170

CORRECTABLE CAUSES

Although most instances of hypertension *cannot* be cured, two of the correctable causes that can be detected by simple physical assessment techniques are (1) coarctation of the aorta and (2) renal artery stenosis.

Coarctation of the aorta

Coarctation of the aorta is a congenital narrowing of a portion of the aorta, usually the last part of the arch. It must be thought of first whenever an elevated BP is found in a child or even a young adult. Early detection is important because of the danger of cerebrovascular accident (from sustained pressure in the arteries of the brain), rupture of the aorta, or heart failure.

Palpation of the peripheral pulses. The principal finding in aortic coarctation is 3+ or 4+ pulses in the upper half of the body and decreased or absent pulses

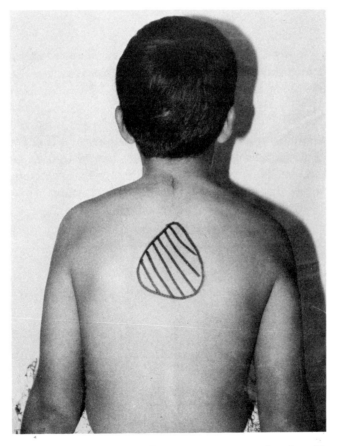

Fig. 39-1. Site of coarctation bruit. Bruit of aortic coarctation is often heard better (or only!) in interscapular area than over anterior chest.

in the lower half. The pulses are also characterized by **radiofemoral delay.** Ordinarily the radial and femoral pulses are felt simultaneously, or perhaps the femoral may be slightly ahead of the radial. However, in coarctation, the femoral pulse falls behind the radial pulse.

Blood pressure readings in the extremities. Ordinarily, blood pressures taken in the legs are slightly higher than those taken in the arms. In measuring blood pressures in the legs, one listens over the popliteal area with the client lying down. In coarctation the blood pressures in the arms are elevated and those in the legs are normal or low.

Systolic bruit. Coarctation produces a systolic crescendo-decrescendo bruit that, if present, is usually well heard over the base of the heart. A portion of this bruit is accounted for by the increased blood flow through the surrounding collateral arterial vessels that form in response to the constriction, and this phenomenon explains why in many instances the bruit is heard best **over the back** (Fig. 39-1).

Renal artery stenosis

Renal artery stenosis is the most common cause of correctable hypertension, and it may produce a systolic bruit in the periumbilical region of the upper abdomen, near the affected artery.

CONGESTIVE HEART FAILURE

One of the major complications in high blood pressure is CHF. After a time the heart begins to fail in its ability to propel blood beyond the peripheral arteriolar constriction, and the client experiences the early dyspneic symptoms of CHF. An S_3 may develop, and this sound may appear before any symptom or any other sign manifests itself.

EXERCISE (*see Appendix E for answers*)

1. Hypertension should be considered whenever a loud _____ sound is auscultated.

2. A characteristic of coarctation of the aorta is _____ delay.

3. In hypertension, auscultating a _____ heart sound may mean moderate-to-severe high BP, but a _____ sound implies CHF.

4. The _____ component of S_2 is responsible for the loud second sound in hypertension.

5. Using the word "high" or "low," describe the pulses one would expect to find in coarctation of the aorta:

    a. Femoral: _____

b. Carotid: ―――――――――――――――――――――

c. Radial: ―――――――――――――――――――――

d. DP: ―――――――――――――――――――――

6. The earliest auscultatory sign of LVH in hypertension is a ――――――― heart sound.
7. When the aortic valve leaflets close with unusual force as a result of the increased

 blood pressure in the aorta, a loud ―――― is produced.
8. Which client is likely to have coarctation of the aorta?

	Client A	Client B
Carotid	4+	1+
Brachial	3+	1+
Radial	3+	1+
Femoral	1+	1+
Popliteal	0	0
DP	1+	1+
PT	0	0

9. Which is an abnormal finding indicative of coarctation of the aorta (*check one*)?
 A. Radial pulsation before femoral
 B. Femoral pulsation before radial
10. A systolic crescendo-decrescendo bruit heard in the upper abdomen may be the result of (*check one*):
 A. CHF
 B. LVH
 C. Coarctation of the aorta
 D. Renal artery stenosis
11. The high arterial pressure in the brain in coarctation of the aorta may lead to

 ――――――――――― accident.
12. The two curable forms of hypertension in this module may both produce

 ――――――――――― crescendo-decrescendo bruits.

MODULE 40

Pulmonary hypertension

Pulmonary hypertension, sometimes called pulmonary heart disease, is an increased pressure in the pulmonary artery. To enable the heart to push blood past this increased resistance in the pulmonary artery, the right ventricle enlarges.

PRINCIPAL CAUSES

Pulmonary hypertension has four principal causes: chronic cor pulmonale, acute cor pulmonale, left-to-right intracardiac shunt, and mitral stenosis.

Chronic cor pulmonale

Chronic cor pulmonale is highly important in that it may constitute perhaps as much as 10% of all heart disease in the United States. The term is defined as enlargement of the right ventricle secondary to chronic obstructive pulmonary disease (COPD). It does not necessarily imply right-sided heart failure, but the danger of the condition is that CHF may occur in the end. In fact, cor pulmonale is frequently not recognized until the right ventricle has failed.

Acute cor pulmonale

The term "acute cor pulmonale" is synonymous with "pulmonary embolism." In this condition the thrombi destroy the pulmonary vascular bed. The right side of the heart must then work harder to pump blood through the remaining vascular bed, resulting in right ventricular failure.

Left-to-right intracardiac shunt

In left-to-right intracardiac shunt, a type of noncyanotic congenital heart defect (Module 42: Cardiovascular Assessment in Children), blood is shunted into the pulmonary circulation, causing increased blood flow through the pulmonary artery and the lungs. The pulmonary artery sometimes responds to this extra flow by constricting actively, even to the point that the pulmonary artery pressure may become higher than the systemic blood pressure, in which case the shunt will reverse, resulting in central cyanosis. (See Module 3: Some Important Physical Signs in Heart Disease). To force blood through the narrowed pulmonary artery, the right ventricle hypertrophies.

Mitral stenosis

In some persons with mitral stenosis, for unknown reasons, the pulmonary artery actively constricts. Once again, the result is RVH.

MAJOR PHYSICAL FINDINGS

The major physical findings in pulmonary hypertension of any cause are (1) increased P_2, (2) right-sided S_4, (3) systolic ejection click, (4) systolic ejection murmur, (5) parasternal lift, (6) large A wave, and (7) signs of right-sided heart failure.

Increased P_2

The elevated pressure in the pulmonary artery causes the pulmonic valve leaflets to snap shut with unusual force, giving rise to a loud P_2. This sound, which is perhaps the earliest sign of pulmonary hypertension, may be palpable in the pulmonic area.

Right-sided S_4

As the right ventricle begins to hypertrophy, an S_4 will be produced. Listen to the right of the apex, close to the sternum, for this sound.

Systolic ejection click

The RVH may forcefully open the pulmonic valve, producing a systolic ejection click that can be heard at the pulmonic area (Module 26: Clicks).

Systolic ejection murmur

The RVH may propel a forceful bolus of blood through the perhaps constricted pulmonary artery, generating a crescendo-decrescendo murmur heard in the pulmonic area.

Parasternal lift

For a discussion of parasternal lift, see Module 6: Palpation.

Large A wave

In pulmonary hypertension the increased pressure in the pulmonary artery causes resistance to the outflow of blood from the right ventricle. Pressure backs up through the ventricle so that the right atrium encounters resistance when it attempts to empty itself into the ventricle. The increased pressure during atrial contraction is reflected in the jugular venous pulse as a prominent A wave (Module 10: Venous Pulse).

Signs of right-sided heart failure

When the right ventricle no longer is able to overcome the resistance created by the increased pulmonary artery pressure, it begins to fail. Signs of CHF can then be discerned (Module 37: Congestive Heart Failure), especially a right-sided S_3, which is heard best at the same location as a right-sided S_4.

EXERCISE *(see Appendix E for answers)*

1. Pulmonary hypertension is an elevated pressure in the pulmonary _____ .

2. Chronic cor pulmonale means enlargement of the right ventricle as a result of _____ .

3. In left-to-right shunts the pulmonary artery may respond to its increased load by constricting. If the pulmonary artery pressure exceeds that in the systemic side of the circulation, the shunt will reverse, resulting in central _____ .

4. The earliest sign of pulmonary heart disease is probably an accentuated _____ .

5. Check the signs one might expect to find in pulmonary hypertension:
   A. Pulsation in the 5-LICS just lateral to the MCL
   B. S_4 heard best at the apex
   C. Palpable P_2
   D. Pulsation in the 4-LICS to the left of the sternum
   E. Prominent diastolic jugular venous pulsation

6. If failure of the right ventricle should eventuate from pulmonary heart disease, one of the first signs would be a right-sided _____ heart sound, best heard close to the sternal border.

MODULE 41

Myocardial infarction

The parameters of assessment in myocardial infarction (MI) are (1) decreased heart sounds, (2) presence of an S_4, (3) signs of CHF, (4) increased or displaced apex beat, (5) systolic murmurs, and (6) pericardial friction rub.

DECREASED HEART SOUNDS

During an acute infarction the first and second sounds are usually fainter than normal, often taking on a ticktack quality. The normal volume of the heart sounds is regained as the heart begins to recover.

PRESENCE OF AN S_4

The finding of a fourth sound is always presumed to be pathological in the client with MI. Although an S_4 may normally occur in a person over the age of 50 years, it is known that 40% to 80% of MI victims develop an S_4 at some point in the acute phase of their illness. In the client over 50 years of age in whom an S_4 was not known prior to the MI, it may possibly disappear altogether as healing takes place. If the client is known to have had an S_4 on previous physical examinations, the sound is not likely to disappear after the infarction, but it can be observed for changes in intensity and proximity to S_1. If there is an acute infarction, the S_4 may become louder and the distance between S_4 and S_1 may widen. As the condition of the client improves, it can be expected that the S_4 will decrease in intensity and move closer to S_1 (near the range of a split first sound).

The appearance of an S_4 in MI is caused by increased tension on the left ventricular wall resulting from ischemic changes in the infarcted muscle tissue. The same phenomenon can be seen in an attack of angina in which an S_4 can be heard during the acute episode but disappears after the attack is over. If further stiffening should occur, as when the ventricle dilates and hypertrophies because of CHF, the fourth sound may disappear and be replaced by an S_3, or the S_3 may appear in addition to the S_4, producing a quadruple rhythm that may then progress to a summation gallop. As the damaged myocardium recuperates and the CHF resolves, the S_3 may disappear and the S_4 may then reappear. As the infarction continues to heal, the S_4 may ultimately fade and perhaps disappear entirely.

SIGNS OF CHF

Congestive failure is second only to electrical rhythm disturbances as a complication of MI. Early detection and treatment of CHF is therefore frequently crucial. Since MI in the vast majority of cases affects the left ventricle, one should be especially alert for symptoms and signs of left-sided failure (Module 37: Congestive Heart Failure). Of particular importance is the third heart sound, which may well be the first and only sign of failure—its mere presence is often sufficient cause to begin diuretic or other drug therapy for CHF.

INCREASED OR DISPLACED APEX BEAT

Whenever a sustained or ectopic PMI is encountered in someone with an MI, three possibilities as to its origin should be borne in mind: the MI itself, ventricular aneurysm, and hypertrophy.

The MI itself

The ischemic area of the heart muscle is somewhat stiffened and lags behind the rest of the ventricular wall during contractile movements. As a result the apex beat may appear sustained or displaced or both. Displacement of the apex beat in MI is usually inward, at a site closer to the sternal border than usual (as may also be noted during an acute attack of angina).

Ventricular aneurysm

If the inward displacement of the PMI persists after healing of the infarction has begun (more than a few days), or if the area of this ectopic pulsation increases in size or force, the reason may be that an aneurysm has formed in the area of the ventricle weakened by the MI.

Hypertrophy

LVH is likely if the PMI is displaced in an outward or a downward direction, or in both directions. The two most common causes of LVH in someone with MI are CHF and hypertension. Occasionally, an aneurysm located right at the apex can produce a similar displacement of the PMI.

SYSTOLIC MURMURS

The systolic murmurs occurring in myocardial infarction are caused either by mitral regurgitation or by rupture of the ventricular septum.

Mitral regurgitation

It is estimated that perhaps as many as 50% of all persons with MI develop a murmur of MR at some time during the course of their illness. The three usual causes are papillary muscle dysfunction, papillary muscle rupture, and CHF.

Papillary muscle dysfunction. If the infarcted area touches the base of one of the papillary muscles (a common occurrence in MI), it may fail to contract properly, allowing one of the mitral valve leaflets to remain open during systole. The result is a soft (grade 1 or 2/4) murmur that occupies part or all of systole and is heard best at the apex. This type of MR is most likely to be heard early in the MI. If the ischemia in the papillary muscle is mild, it may respond to conservative medical treatment, in which case the murmur will cease. While it is present, however, the murmur should be monitored closely because of the danger of rupture of the papillary muscle.

Papillary muscle rupture. Rupture may occur with or without evidence of previous papillary muscle dysfunction. Papillary rupture is heralded by a loud, **holo**systolic murmur because the leaflet attached to the ruptured muscle is wide open as the ventricle contracts. If there had been previous papillary dysfunction, it would be noted that the systolic murmur dramatically intensifies and becomes longer when the rupture occurs. Since the left side of the heart seldom has time to adapt to the sudden increase in the pressure load, frank pulmonary edema and death may quickly ensue.

Presence of CHF. In advanced failure the left ventricle dilates to such an extent that the mitral valve ring stretches enough to spread the leaflets apart. Blood thus leaks backward across the valve into the left atrium, producing a *functional* murmur of MR. This soft murmur occupies part or all of systole. As the CHF responds to therapy and the mitral leaflets once again are able to shut securely, the murmur disappears.

Rupture of the ventricular septum

Another dreaded complication of MI is rupture of the ventricular septum. It is likely to occur in those infarctions involving the septum (such infarctions are common) and, in effect, creates an artifical VSD. High-risk surgery was formerly the only treatment, but recent advances such as vasodilator therapy and counterpulsation by intra-aortic balloon have made nonsurgical treatment possible. However, the success of these measures depends on prompt detection and initiation of therapy. If one is standing beside the bed when septal rupture occurs, it can sometimes be heard with the unaided ear. It produces a loud holosystolic murmur exactly like that of papillary muscle rupture. A point of distinction between the two types of rupture is that in septal rupture the jet produced by blood gushing through the hole travels directly forward, striking the lower left chest wall and giving rise to a thrill that is easily palpable. However, whether a thrill is present or not, it must be emphasized that the discovery of **any loud systolic murmur in someone with an MI is an urgent event.** Those caring for clients with MI would do well to commit to memory the following rhyme:

Loud murmur found
'Twixt first and second sound
Warns of rupture
In cardiac structure.

PERICARDIAL FRICTION RUB

Pericarditis is a common complication of MI, occurring in as many as 16% of all persons with this condition. The area of infarcted tissue inflames the overlying pericardium. The two layers of the pericardium become roughened and as they rub against each other give rise to the friction sounds. The sounds are generally heard best at the lower end of the sternum and are not necessarily associated with chest pain. Pericardial rubs usually begin to be heard on the second or third day after the MI and last two or three days. They may also be heard in **postmyocardial infarction syndrome** (Dressler's syndrome), which is a brief flare-up of pericarditis that occurs in a small percentage of MI cases some weeks or months after the infarction. It is thought to be an autoimmune reaction to the necrotic tissue. The appearance of a friction rub in the MI client who is on anticoagulants warrants temporarily withholding these drugs because of the danger of precipitating hemopericardium and cardiac tamponade.

EXERCISE *(see Appendix E for answers)*

1. The finding of a _____ heart sound in a person with MI is always presumed to be abnormal.

2. The appearance of a _____ heart sound in a client with MI is considered to be evidence of CHF.

3. Describe the most likely direction of displacement of the PMI in the following conditions, using the word "inward" or "outward":

   a. MI of the anterior heart surface: _____

   b. Aneurysm at the apex: _____

   c. Hypertrophy due to hypertension: _____

   d. Left-sided CHF: _____

4. You are assessing a client with MI. Yesterday an S_4 was present, but the interval between it and the following S_1 seemed spacious. Today the S_4 is of the same intensity, but it is so close to S_1 that the two sounds almost blend together. Your assessment is that the client's condition is *(check one)*:
   A. About the same
   B. Better
   C. Worse

5. Describe the most likely intensity of the systolic murmur in the following conditions, using the word "soft" or "loud":

   a. Functional MR due to CHF: _____

   b. Papillary muscle rupture: _____

   c. Papillary muscle dysfunction: _____

   d. Rupture of the ventricular septum: _____

6. Mr. Carr D. Eck, your next-door neighbor, calls you because of severe chest pain. While waiting for the ambulance to arrive, you examine him. Check which of the following findings favor a possible MI:
   A. Loud first sound
   B. Loud fourth sound
   C. Decreased first and second sounds
   D. PMI in the 5-LICS at the mitral area
   E. PMI in the 5-LICS at the tricuspid area

MODULE 42

Cardiovascular assessment in children

The same principles of assessment that apply to adults, as given in the rest of the text, generally apply to children as well. Examination features unique to children are set forth in this module. In pediatric cardiovascular assessment there are two additional examination tools that should be employed liberally to facilitate accurate gathering of data: the nipple and the lollipop. (Fig. 42-1). The cardinal rule for assessing the heart in children states: **Always examine in both lying and sitting positions.**

INSPECTION FOR CENTRAL CYANOSIS

Central cyanosis is always a red flag that calls for pediatrician consultation (Module 3: Some Important Physical Signs in Heart Disease). It is normal in some babies only during the first week of life, and then only when the infant is crying vigorously. When normal in the postnatal period, it is due to **patent foramen ovale.** The foramen ovale closes immediately after birth as the intracardiac pressure changes cause a vane to cover the opening. In most people the vane later adheres permanently and the hole fills in with fibrous tissue (although slight patency without symptoms may persist into adulthood and can be found in as many as 25% of normal adults). Even if the foramen does not become permanently sealed, the vane acts as a one-way valve and thus remains closed unless pressure in the right atrium overcomes that in the left (which, after birth, occurs only during crying and forces unoxygenated blood into the oxygenated blood circulating through the left side of the heart). Furthermore, as the circulatory readjustments initiated by the birth process are completed, it becomes more and more difficult for the right atrial pressure to exceed that of the left atrium; this kind of cyanosis is never normal beyond the first few days.

In newborn infants it is crucial to distinguish between peripheral and central cyanosis. In the neonate, peripheral cyanosis is invariably normal and occurs for two reasons: (1) The normally high hematocrit of the newborn "thickens" the blood and slows oxygen transport to the tissues, and (2) the thin skin permits easier cooling and makes the deeper vascular beds more visible.

Central cyanosis is almost always the result of a congenital **right-to-left shunt** in the heart (venous blood entering the arterial circulation, or V⟶A). Depending on the type and severity of the congenital anomaly, it may be noticed immediately

Fig. 42-1. Two additional "tools" to be included in the examination kit of everyone who assesses children.

after birth or may be first seen months or even years later. Central cyanosis is not usually noticed by the parents, but if it is, it is most likely to be seen during feeding, when the infant begins to turn blue and struggle for breath (a form of DOE). Failure to thrive or gain weight, poor general physical development, and frequent upper respiratory infections are other significant clues to the presence of a V⟶A shunt. If the cyanosis is mild, the body may attempt to compensate by producing an excess of red blood cells, which may give a deceptive "rosy-cheeked" appearance to the child. In the older child, **clubbing** of the fingers is a valuable sign that points to the possibility of congenital cyanotic heart disease. The child with a cyanotic defect may first present because the parents have noticed that the child interrupts play to rest in a squatting position. This maneuver increases resistance to the venous blood trying to enter the arterial system through the shunt.

PALPATION

Although the signs discussed below are grouped under the heading of "palpation," they may be first detected at inspection, and they also may be confirmed by accompanying auscultatory findings.

Rhythm

Occasional premature beats are not uncommon in childhood and are generally of no concern. The so-called **sinus arrhythmia** is simply an increased heart rate during inspiration and is entirely normal in young adults and children. It is so marked in many young children that the heart rate may double that in expiration, giving the impression of a severe arrhythmia. Doubt can easily be removed by having the child hold the breath for a few moments, which will make the variability disappear.

Apex beat

After a child reaches approximately the age of 7 years, the PMI assumes its "adult" location in the 5-LICS just medial to or at the MCL. Before this age the PMI is located in the 4-LICS and may normally be found up to 1.25 cm ($^1/_2$ in) *outside* the MCL. In infancy the apex beat may even be found as high as the 3-LICS—again, outside the MCL. If the PMI is located on the right side of the chest, suspect dextrocardia.

Sternal bulging

Hypertrophy of the right ventricle causes a deformity in which the lower end of the sternum and the surrounding ribs project forward.

AUSCULTATION
Splitting of S_1

Splitting of S_1 is uncommon (usually narrow when encountered) but is not abnormal. It is perhaps more common in children than adults.

Splitting of S_2

The S_2 is universally split in inspiration if the heart rate is not too rapid; a crisp, perfectly single S_2 in infancy is indicative of congenital cyanotic heart disease. The P_2 may normally be louder than A_2 in children. Splitting of S_2 in expiration in children who are lying down is not necessarily considered abnormal unless it persists in the upright position.

Presence of S_3

One third of all children and adolescents develop a loud third sound that disappears by early adulthood. This fact makes it difficult at times to distinguish a physiological S_3 from a pathological third sound, which indicates heart failure, but palpation can sometimes enable the examiner to differentiate the two. A physiological third sound can never be felt, but a pathological S_3 can cause the three beats to become palpable at the apex.

Murmurs

All murmurs encountered in early infancy are to be suspected as a sign of congenital heart disease. The vast majority of murmurs encountered in children who have reached the toddler stage are innocent, but if a murmur is combined with a fever in the kindergarten or school-age child, think of rheumatic fever. Remember:

$$ⓜ + \text{Fever} + \text{Child} \rightarrow \text{RF}$$

The four common types of innocent childhood murmurs are listed below in order of prominence. They usually occur between the ages of 2 and 7 years. Note that with the exception of the venous hum they are all systolic, short (i.e., *not* pansystolic), soft, and well localized (i.e., do not radiate), and that S_1 and S_2 are distinctly heard and are always normal. To further establish the innocence of a murmur, (1) take BP reading in the arms and legs and (2) listen over the interscapular area. The reason for this additional examination is that the murmur of coarctation of the aorta sometimes *sounds* innocent because it is a soft systolic murmur that is usually heard well at the pulmonic area and that closely resembles the pulmonic ejection murmur (see outline below). If coarctation is present, the murmur may be heard louder over the back, and the blood pressures in the legs will be lower than those in the arms.

1. Vibratory murmur
   a. Short but sometimes loud
   b. Localized to LLSB
   c. Described as musical, squeaky, twangy, or moaning
2. Venous hum
   a. Continuous through systole and diastole, thus covering the heart sounds
   b. Caused by rapid flow through the jugular veins
   c. Heard just above or just below the clavicle—may be right, left, or bilateral but is most often right and supraclavicular (Fig. 42-2)
   d. Decreases in loudness, or ceases if jugular blood flow is decreased by lying down, twisting the neck, or compressing the jugular
   e. In populations composed mostly of healthy young adults (e.g., college, military), called "30-30" bruit, meaning that up to 30% of adults under 30 years of age may have it; nearly all pregnant women affected
3. Pulmonic ejection murmur
   a. Soft and blowing
   b. Localized to pulmonic area
4. Supraclavicular (carotid) bruit (Fig. 42-2)
   a. Produced by turbulence of blood passing through subclavian, innominate, and carotid arteries
   b. Systolic crescendo-decrescendo bruit
   c. Also heard in some normal young adults

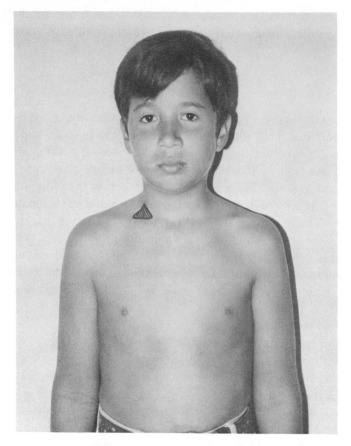

Fig. 42-2. Site of venous hum and supraclavicular bruit.

 d. Heard just above clavicle—most often on the right but occasionally bilateral

 e. Ceases when the shoulders are pulled back (hyperextended) as far as possible

ASSESSMENT IN CONGENITAL HEART DISEASE

The incidence of cardiac birth defects is six to eight per 1,000 live births and as such is a significant public health problem. In taking the mother's prenatal and perinatal history, be sure to ask whether anyone else in the family has had congenital malformations of any kind (not only cardiac) and whether the mother was exposed to viral infections such as German measles (rubella) or to any drugs at all during the first trimester. Although most cardiac defects are associated with murmurs, the murmur may not be present at birth and may only develop days or weeks later, if at all. Thus the examiner must avoid overemphasizing the pres-

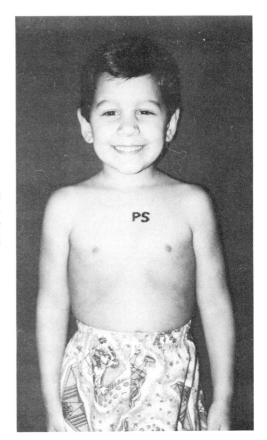

Fig. 42-3. Auscultatory site for pulmonic stenosis. At this location, listen for (1) ejection murmur, (2) ejection click, (3) widely split S_2 due to delayed P_2, and (4) decreased P_2.

ence or absence of murmurs in babies but rather should build reliance on other clinical features as well. Congenital cardiac disease is divided into three broad categories:

1. *Stenotic lesions* —three most common
    a. Coarctation of the aorta (Module 39: Systemic Hypertension)
    b. Pulmonic stenosis (PS) (Fig. 42-3)
        (1) Common—10% of all congenital heart disease
        (2) Development of RVH—an attempt to overcome resistance of stenosed valve
        (3) Loud, harsh ejection murmur and thrill over the pulmonic area or Erb's point
        (4) P_2 may be soft, absent, or delayed (S_2 widely split)
        (5) May be an ejection click in mild-to-moderate disease and right-sided S_4 in severe disease
    c. Aortic stenosis

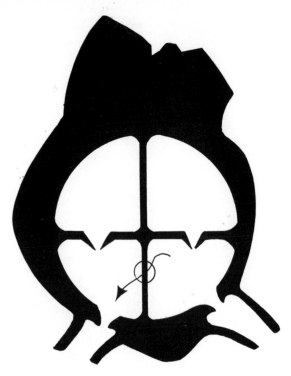

Fig. 42-4. Ventricular septal defect (VSD). Flow through the hole is in direction of arrow. If hole is small, turbulent flow is produced, generating a murmur that lasts through ventricular contraction (pansystolic) and a thrill that is palpable over area of right ventricle. If defect is large, no murmur is produced.

2. *Left-to-right shunts* (arterial-to-venous, or A⟶V; acyanotic)
   a. Ventricular septal defect (VSD) (Fig. 42-4)
      (1) Most common congenital lesion
      (2) Usually small, and closes spontaneously before adulthood
      (3) Holosystolic murmur, often harsh or blowing, usually loud and accompanied by a thrill
      (4) Murmur heard best at LLSB (Fig. 42-5). (The innocent vibratory murmur is also heard at this site, but the key to distinguishing it from VSD is the **holosystolic** nature of the latter murmur, which may cover A_2 and obscure it.)
   b. Atrial septal defect (ASD) (Fig. 42-6)
      (1) Defect so large that it does not produce a murmur (generates no turbulence)
      (2) Flow murmurs at tricuspid and pulmonic valves, especially the latter, produced by increased flow through the right side of the heart

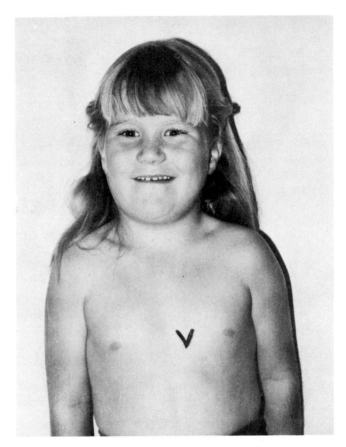

Fig. 42-5. Site of VSD murmur. In a VSD the jet of blood strikes anterior wall of right ventricle so that the murmur (and thrill, if present) can be found at area adjacent to lower left sternal edge.

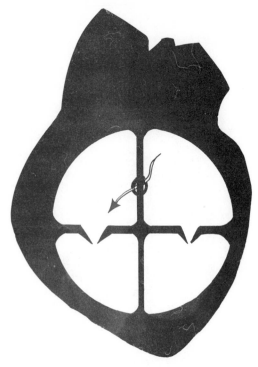

Fig. 42-6. Atrial septal defect (ASD). Flow through hole is in direction of arrow.

        (a) Tricuspid flow murmur—an early diastolic murmur heard over tricuspid area

        (b) Pulmonic flow murmur—similar to innocent pulmonic ejection murmur described earlier; key distinguishing signs are **wide, fixed splitting** of S_2 in ASD, which persists when the child is sitting upright, and signs of RVH

     (3) ASD virtually ruled out if the ECG is normal

  c. Patent ductus arteriosus (PDA) (Fig. 42-7)

     (1) Murmur heard best just under clavicle or in pulmonic area (Fig. 42-8)

     (2) Continuous, **machinery-like** murmur that is seldom mistaken for anything else (Fig. 42-9)

 3. *Right-to-left shunts* (venous-to-arterial, or V⟶A; cyanotic) (The key sign of the major cyanotic conditions is a clear, crisp, sometimes accentuated, **single second sound.**)

  a. Tetralogy of Fallot (Fig. 42-10)

     (1) Most common cyanotic lesion

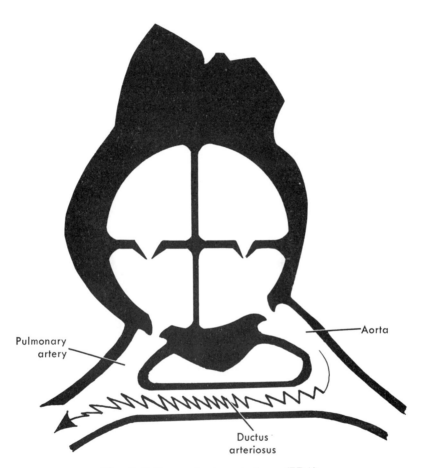

Fig. 42-7. Patent ductus arteriosus (PDA).

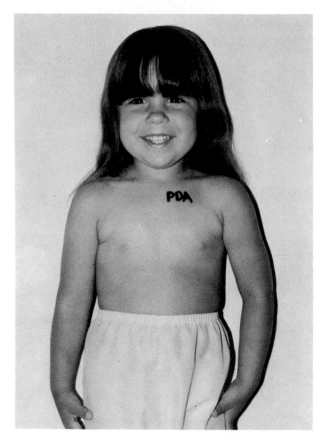

Fig. 42-8. Site of murmur of PDA.

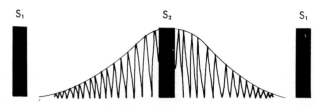

Fig. 42-9. Continuous murmur of PDA builds to a peak around second heart sound.

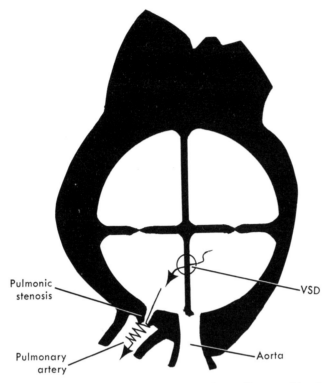

Fig. 42-10. Tetralogy of Fallot (TF). This condition is basically a combination of pulmonic stenosis plus a VSD. Note that the aorta overrides both left and right ventricles. Because the right ventricle has to work hard to overcome resistance posed by PS, a parasternal tap of RVH is a prominent finding in this condition.

(2) Lay term—"blue baby disease"
(3) Basically a combination of PS and a VSD
(4) VSD so large that it does not produce a murmur
(5) Murmur of PS
(6) Single S_2, the result of loss of P_2 because of PS
    b. Transposition of the great vessels
        (1) Aorta arising from *right* ventricle; pulmonary artery arising from *left* ventricle
        (2) Venous and arterial circulations totally separate from each other
        (3) Immediate surgery necessary for survival after birth unless there is another defect that can provide a communication between the two circulations
        (4) One or more left-to-right shunts (which permit life until corrective surgery is performed) also present at birth in many cases
        (5) Murmurs not typical; if present, result from coexisting left-to-right defect (VSD, ASD, or PDA)

MODULE 43

Review two

1. The most common cause of a friction rub is —————————————————

   ———————————————————————.

2. The most commonly encountered friction rub is a biphasic rub. List the audible components:

   a. ————————————————————————————————

   b. ————————————————————————————————

3. Mrs. Tammy Ponada is on permanent oral anticoagulant therapy for recurrent thrombophlebitis of the legs. She was driving to work this morning when she was involved in an accident that threw her chest against the steering wheel. She comes to the ED complaining of pain in the anterior chest, and while auscultating her precordium, you note a loud friction rub. Since you are concerned about the possibility of a pericardial effusion that may impede the contractions of the heart, you quickly assess other parameters. If Mrs. Ponada's heart were being constricted by an effusion, the most sensitive indicator would be ————————————————————.

4. Check the correct statement(s):
   A. Clicks are always pathological but never serious.
   B. Ejection clicks are heard in systole and nonejection clicks in diastole.
   C. A split S_1 auscultated in the tricuspid area or LLSB in reality is most likely an S_1 plus an ejection click.
   D. Clicks are heard only in systole.

5. Check the signs that are produced by turbulence of the blood flow:
   A. Bruits
   B. Rubs
   C. Murmurs
   D. Crackles
   E. Thrills

6. Check which of the following murmurs may be innocent:
   A. Early systolic murmur
   B. Early diastolic murmur
   C. Long systolic murmur that obscures S_1
   D. Loud crescendo-decrescendo systolic murmur
   E. Short, soft murmur heard between S_2 and S_1

NOTE: See Appendix E for answers.

194

7. An ejection murmur caused by hyperkinetic circulation across a normal valve is often referred to as a _____ murmur.

8. Describe the grades of the 4-step scale of murmur intensity:

    a. Grade 1: _____

    b. Grade 2: _____

    c. Grade 3: _____

    d. Grade 4: _____

9. Fever + (m) ⟶ _____ .

10. Fever + (m) + Child ⟶ _____ .

11. You are attending Scarlet Reumer, a 7-year-old girl in the acute phase of RF. Since you began to take care of her, a murmur has been continually present, indicating that the disease process is probably remaining at the level of the endocardium. You wish to be alert for the spread of the pathological process to other structures, the most untoward instance of which would be signaled by the appearance of a

    _____ .

12. Murmurs tend to be propagated in the direction of _____

    _____ and therefore are often heard loudest _____

    from their points of origin.

13. Match the physical findings in column A with the diseases in column B:

A	**B**
a. Soft ejection murmur confined to aortic area	A. Aortic stenosis
b. Rise of carotid pulse is prolonged	B. Aortic regurgitation
c. Harsh ejection murmur heard all over chest	C. Aortic sclerosis
d. Faint early diastolic murmur	
e. Strong, jerking radial pulse	
f. BP, 110/95	
g. BP, 180/55	

14. List the two hallmark signs of MS:

    a. _____

    b. _____

15. The _____ quality of a murmur heard at the apex is the tip-off to MS.

16. The murmur of MS is a sound of _____ pitch and therefore is heard best with the _____ of the stethoscope.

17. The most common cause of MR is _____ in which the dilation of the left ventricle stretches open the mitral valve ring, permitting backward flow of blood.

18. You are auscultating at the apex and hear an extra sound before the midpoint of diastole. To help you distinguish between OS and an S_3, you recall that firm pressure with the diaphragm will block out or reduce an _____ .

19. Your client, Mr. M., complains of being out of breath after walking only two blocks. During the course of examining Mr. M., you begin auscultation at the aortic area and notice right away that the first sound is louder than the second. This finding leads you to suspect *(check one)*:
    A. Floppy mitral valve syndrome
    B. Mitral stenosis
    C. Mitral regurgitation
    D. Aortic valvular disease of some kind

20. Check the following statement(s) that describe the murmur of MR:
    A. Radiates to carotids
    B. Localized to apex
    C. Radiates to axilla
    D. Diamond-shaped
    E. Rectangular
    F. Decrescendo

21. The hallmark of the billowing mitral leaflet syndrome is a _____

    systolic _____ .

22. A murmur of _____ is sometimes heard in the floppy mitral valve syndrome.

23. Since congestion always occurs rearward from the failing ventricle in CHF, we can

    anticipate that edema in left ventricular failure will occur in the _____ .

24. The earliest auscultatory finding of CHF is *(check one)*:
    A. Rales
    B. Wheezes
    C. Expiratory split of S_2
    D. Murmur of MR
    E. S_4
    F. S_3

25. All that wheezes is not _____ .

26. Classify the following signs and symptoms as "right" or "left" to indicate the failing ventricle:

    a. Indigestion: _____

    b. Crepitations: _____

    c. Difficulty putting shoes on: _____

    d. Nightmares, trouble sleeping, sleeping propped up on two pillows: _____

    e. Dry cough at night, especially in left lateral decubitus position: _____

    f. S_3 midway between apex and LLSB: _____

    g. Urinating several times in the middle of the night: _____

    h. Confusion: _____

    i. Eyeballs pulsating in systole: _____

27. Aortic aneurysms often produce abnormal _____ that are usually seen in the 2- and 3-RICS and the suprasternal notch.

28. Whenever a high blood pressure reading is found in a child or young adult, the curable condition known as _____ should be considered first.

29. If, after placing the stethoscope on the client's chest, you hear an unusually loud S_2 (in any location), you should immediately suspect _____

_____ .

30. Select the findings that could be expected in someone with renal artery stenosis:.
    A. Decreased femoral pulses
    B. S_4
    C. Parasternal lift
    D. Systolic bruit in the interscapular area
    E. Systolic bruit in the periumbilical area

31. In hypertension, if the left ventricle begins to fail in its ability to pump blood past the constricted peripheral arterioles, an _____ may develop.

32. The earliest palpable sign of LVH in systemic hypertension is an apex beat of increased _____ .

33. To enable the heart to push blood past the increased resistance in the pulmonary artery in pulmonary hypertension, the _____ enlarges.

34. Just as the elevated aortic pressure in arterial hypertension causes the aortic valve leaflets to close forcefully, producing a loud A_2, so pulmonary hypertension may similarly give rise to a loud _____ , which may sometimes be palpated in the _____ area.

35. Conditions in which pulmonary hypertension is a pathophysiological mechanism give rise to a right-sided _____ .

36. In pulmonary hypertension a systolic ejection _____ and _____ can frequently be heard in the pulmonic area.

37. The danger of conditions that feature pulmonary hypertension is that they may lead to failure of the right ventricle which would be heralded by a right-sided _____ .

38. The ischemic area of the heart muscle in an acute MI may give rise to a _____ heart sound.

39. Displacement of the apex beat early in MI is not uncommon, but if the beat persists in its ectopic location, the reason may be that a ventricular _____ has formed.

40. In an acute MI, a soft systolic murmur of MR is most likely due to _____ in the early phase, whereas later on, such a murmur is more commonly the functional murmur of _____ .

41. A loud systolic murmur with MI indicates _____ of a cardiac structure.

42. Central _____ is normal only during the first few days of life when the baby cries lustily.

43. Doubt about whether a child has a pathological arrhythmia or merely sinus arrhythmia can be resolved by having the child _____.

44. You are examining a 5-year-old boy named Ricky. Check the findings that would be abnormal for a child of his age:
    A. Loud P_2
    B. PMI in 4-LICS to left of MCL
    C. Fine splitting of S_1
    D. Third heart sound
    E. Localized musical murmur at LLSB
    F. None of the above

45. A crisp, single S_2 in infancy suggests congenital _____ heart disease.

46. Sandra, a 4-year-old girl, is heard to have a soft, short, crescendo-decrescendo murmur that seems to be localized to the pulmonic area. The S_1 and S_2 are well heard and are normal, and the initial impression is that the murmur is innocent. When the examiner listens over the back, a similar but louder murmur is heard. In this situation, however, one would expect BP readings in Sandra's arms to be _____ but those in her legs to be _____ .

47. Check the murmur(s) that is (are) abnormal:
    A. Systolic bruit heard in a 25-year-old pregnant woman in the right supraclavicular area
    B. Continuous bruit heard in a 25-year-old pregnant woman in the right supraclavicular area
    C. Loud, harsh ejection murmur at pulmonic area
    D. Holosystolic murmur at LLSB

48. The key signs of ASD are wide, fixed splitting of S_2, even with the child fully upright, and signs of RVH, such as a parasternal _____ .

49. An infraclavicular, machinery-like, continuous murmur is typical of _____ .

50. The key to distinguishing an innocent vibratory murmur from the murmur of VSD is the _____ nature of the latter.

51. In tetralogy of Fallot, the murmur is produced by the _____ .

52. Identify the following murmurs:
    a. Grade 2/4 low-pitched, rumbling, middiastolic murmur with crescendo accentuation in late diastole, localized to the apex, and heard only with the client in the left lateral decubitus position: _____ .
    b. Grade 4/6 harsh holosystolic murmur heard loudest at the apex and radiating to left axilla: _____ .
    c. Grade 1/4 blowing early diastolic murmur best heard at the aortic area, with the client in the seated flexion position and breath held in full expiration: _____ .

MODULE 44

Case illustration

Mr. A., a 35-year-old junior executive, was brought to the ED because of severe, pressing substernal pain (Fig. 44-1). The pain had begun suddenly about a half-hour earlier while he was doing paperwork at his desk. At first he assumed that the pain was just another instance of heartburn, which he occasionally experienced, even though this time it was intense and had a pressure quality it had never had before. A double dose of his usual antacid provided no relief. When the pain increased and began to radiate down the right arm, he called an ambulance. He later denied shortness of breath, syncope, or palpitations.

After arrival at the hospital, the client was in a state of near panic, weeping, talking incoherently, and hyperventilating. Between gasps he described his pain as follows: "It's like someone was pushing a knife into the center of my chest. It goes up into my shoulder and down the inside of my upper arm like a wire. When it gets to my elbow it crosses over to the outside. Then it feels like electricity running down the outside of my forearm and into my little finger and ring finger." After being placed in one of the treatment bays, Mr. A. began to complain excitedly of numbness and tingling in both hands. An intern pulled the paper bag off the side rail of Mr. A.'s gurney and had him breathe in and out of it several times, which promptly relieved the paresthesia. At this point the intern became convinced that the client was a "crock" who should be given a tranquilizer and sent home. What led the intern to this conclusion was Mr. A.'s agitated behavior, his description of the chest pain as "sharp" and its radiation "like a wire" and "like electricity," the crossing over of the pain to the outside of the arm at the elbow, and most of all, his response to the "paper-bag" trick. The intern explained to one of the nurses that the paresthesia was due to respiratory alkalosis brought on by blowing off excess amounts of carbon dioxide during hyperventilation. Rebreathing CO_2 in the paper bag restored the acid-base balance, causing the paresthesia to disappear. The intern added that this was proof of hyperventilation syndrome, a purely psychogenic disorder. By this time a more experienced emergency physician came on the scene and ordered a stat ECG, which revealed a large myocardial infarction.

Psychosocial assessment, derived mostly from interviews with family members, showed Mr. A. to be a hard-driving, impatient, demanding person who found it difficult to relax. His job involved much pressure to deliver a high volume of work in a small span of time, and although he was heard to complain about this aspect of his work at times, he seemed restless when work demands happened to be slack. His military history disclosed that his four-year term of service was spent entirely in explosive ordnance disposal. Ever since the death of one of his children three months before, he had been spending longer hours on the job. Two weeks before this episode, he had received an offer to take a different type of job in another city for a higher salary, but he was still undecided about whether to accept at the time of admission to the hospital.

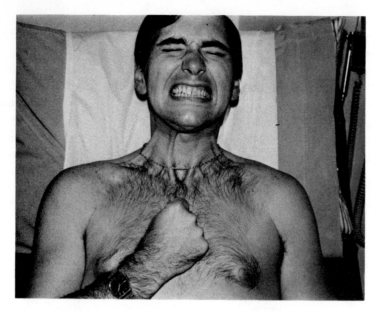

Fig. 44-1. Client describing chest pain in the ED.

DISCUSSION: In this description the four cardinal symptoms of heart disease are touched on, but only chest pain is positive. The five dimensions of pain (PQRST) are all accounted for.

Practitioners are sometimes led astray by presentations of an illness that do not fit the textbook picture of that illness. Although the history given by Mr. A. is not *classic* for myocardial infarction, only one feature of his description is not compatible with that disease, namely, the paresthesia of the hands. Nothing in the rest of his story could legitimately be considered strange for or opposed to an MI. Health care providers seldom fail to pursue infarction when radiation occurs down the left arm, but at times we have been fooled by the less frequent patterns of radiation to both arms and particularly to the right arm alone. As in this illustration, inexperienced interviewers are also commonly misled by failures to appreciate the numerous subjective factors that color the way individuals perceive and interpret pain. The young doctor mislabeled the client's description of pain as sharp simply because Mr. A. had used the word "knife." Actually, many people use the image of a knife to describe the *intensity* of their pain rather than a lancinating quality. Note also that the intern ignored the word **pushing,** which Mr. A. was using to express his experience of pressure. Although the description of the radiation into the arm as being "like a wire" and "like electricity" sounded psychogenic to the intern, many persons may employ the image of a wire in describing any kind of pain that occurs along the length of an extremity as a means of emphasizing its *extensiveness*. In addition, an electricity-like quality is not an uncommon descriptor of any kind of extremity pain that travels "in a current" along a nerve distribution in that extremity (ischemic heart pain follows the ulnar nerve distribution).

Another point of Mr. A.'s history that sounded neurotic to the young doctor was the "switching" of the pain at the elbow from the inside of the upper arm to the outer aspect of the forearm, since the intern had learned in medical school that cardiac pain radiates only down the inner aspect of the arm and never occurs on the outside. However, this is true only if the subject is in the standard anatomical position shown in textbooks (i.e., with the thumb toward the outside). Clients lying on a bed or gurney are most inclined to demonstrate their arm with the hand *pronated* (thumb inward), in which case pain that travels down the ulnar nerve will indeed be understood to "cross over" to the outside at the elbow. Pain or a sensation of weakness in the last two fingers or the little finger alone can occur sometimes as the first manifestation of ischemic heart pain (as happened when the tennis star Arthur Ashe had an MI) or at other times as an extension of the radiation from the upper arm. The physiological explanation for the paresthesia and treatment (rebreathing CO_2) given by the intern are correct, but in this case the hyperventilation is a manifestation of an *appropriate* anxiety state stemming from life-threatening organic injury. Finally, the young physician violated the Cardinal Principle of Chest Pain by disregarding the possibility of an infarction.

Mr. A. demonstrates a marked type A personality pattern. Attributing the chest pain to heartburn despite the fact that it was qualitatively different from his usual bouts of heartburn resulted in a delay of the necessary treatment and is an example of the unhealthy use of denial. His military history consisted of an extremely and chronically stressful assignment of defusing bombs. His present job is high in stress/tension/pressure (STP). There recently has been an enormously stressful change in his life, the death of his child, and even more recently he has been considering two more significant life changes—moving and taking a new job. If Mr. A. had been fortunate enough to receive health care prior to this episode, it would have been prudent to counsel postponement of taking the new job until more time had elapsed to permit adjustment to the first life change.

> Mr. A. is taken to the cardiac care unit, where an initial assessment is made by his coronary nurse. The findings are as follows: temperature—37 C; pulse—92, regular, and force +2; respirations—22; BP—120/65; skin—warm, pink, and dry; heart—PMI located by both inspection and palpation in the 5-LICS halfway between the MCL and the left sternal border, S_1 and S_2 are both distant but otherwise normal, and a faint S_4 is occasionally heard. Soon the morphine and diazepam given in the ED take their full effect, and the client drifts off to sleep.

DISCUSSION: The normal blood pressure, good color, and warm, dry skin are indicators that Mr. A. is not in shock. Although the PMI is located in the normal intercostal space, it is ectopic because it is located closer to the sternal edge than would be expected. Apex beats that are medial to their usual location are most often due to an ischemic area of the myocardium. Thus Mr. A.'s PMI supports the assessment that the client is in the acute phase of an MI. The presence of an S_4 tends to confirm this assessment, since a fourth sound is abnormal in someone of the client's age (recall that an S_4 may be normal in elderly people). The decreased heart sounds and decreased force of the pulse also suggest the acute phase.

> The next morning Mr. A. awakens free of pain and is informed by his physician that he has had an MI. Assessment on the second day shows the following: temperature— 38.3 C; pulse—84, regular, and of normal force; respirations—16; BP—155/90; heart—PMI located in the 5-LICS just inside the MCL, S_1 and S_2 have returned to their full volume, and there is no evidence of a gallop rhythm. The client tells his nurse that 155/90 is his usual blood pressure.

DISCUSSION: The assessment is made that the client is doing well for the second day. His physician upgrades his status from the very serious list to the serious list. The temperature elevation can be attributed to the body's expected response to the area of necrosis in the heart muscle, since a low-grade fever is not an unusual finding in the first few days after an MI. The return of the PMI to its usual location, the disappearance of the S_4, and the return of the heart sounds and pulse to their normal volume are all favorable signs indicating that the acute phase has passed and that healing is beginning to take place. Mr. A.'s statement that 155/90 is his usual blood pressure makes it clear that the previous BP of 120/ 65 was relatively depressed for him and correlates with the decreased pulse force and intensity of heart sounds at that time.

> On the evening of the second day Mr. A. is unchanged except that his temperature has dropped to 37.7 C. The night nurse, making initial assessments after receiving a report, finds Mr. A. awake and does a thorough cardiovascular assessment. The only positive findings are the temperature elevation and a third heart sound. The nurse immediately notifies the house officer, who agrees with the findings and orders intravenous furosemide and digoxin and the insertion of a Swan-Ganz catheter.

DISCUSSION: The nurse has intercepted an early congestive heart failure by detecting an S_3.

> By the morning of the third day the temperature has returned to 37 C. After a night of fitful sleep Mr. A. begins to notice a slight, dry cough. The S_3 is present but is still faint. The PMI is in its normal location and measures 1 to 2 cm, but the nurse who is examining Mr. A. notes that the pulsation seems to stay in contact with the flat of the hand significantly longer than previously. The client's respirations are 18, and he denies shortness of breath.

DISCUSSION: The return of the temperature to normal simply signifies the clearing of the febrile response to the myocardial necrosis. It cannot be deduced from this that the client's condition is improving. In fact, it is worsening because his CHF is advancing. The cough, which at this stage is easy to ignore or attribute to a virus, is consistent with an early CHF. The PMI is in the usual location and is normal in size, but its sustained quality favors enlargement of the heart. The assessment is made that the client is not responding to therapy for the CHF.

Late on the third day, the evening nurse auscultates Mr. A.'s lungs and hears a few fine inspiratory crackles at both bases. The respirations are still 18, and there is no dyspnea apart from the cough, which is about the same. The S_3 is still present and is noticeably louder. During the course of the night the client becomes frankly dyspneic even though resting in high Fowler's position, and his oxygen unit must be turned up high to keep cyanosis from appearing on his lips and fingernails. Percussion reveals dullness at the lung bases, and coarse crackles can be heard up to the middle zone of the lungs. By the fourth day the PMI can be palpated just outside the MCL and can be seen in *two* intercostal spaces.

DISCUSSION: The advent of the crackles and the dullness at the lung bases signify pulmonary edema, and these are relatively late signs of left-sided failure. In some patients, as with Mr. A., they may be present even though the client experiences neither subjective nor objective respiratory distress in early pulmonary edema. As the lungs fill with fluid and the level of crackles rises, however, frank respiratory distress eventually becomes inevitable. The coarse, ascending crackles, the loud S_3, the peripheral cyanosis, and the development of a leftward heave are signs that the left ventricular failure has continued to worsen. Mr. A.'s name is once again added to the very serious list.

By the morning of the fourth day, Mr. A. is sleeping all the time. He can be aroused if his name is called loudly, but he immediately goes back to sleep. His cough is now productive of pink-tinged sputum, but there is no fever. The nurse, while taking his blood pressure, notes that after the first few beats are heard, the rate of the beats suddenly doubles. An S_4 can now be heard in addition to the S_3, giving a quadruple rhythm, and a faint holosystolic murmur can be heard at the PMI. It is noticed that the neck veins are engorged when Mr. A. is in high Fowler's position. When the nurses turn him, they discover pitting edema over the sacrum. The area of liver dullness is percussed to 14 cm in the MCL. That afternoon the intern who admitted Mr. A. happens to be on duty. The intern examines the client and then announces that Mr. A.'s condition has slightly improved, the quadruple rhythm having returned to triple rhythm. The attending nurse also examines Mr. A. and agrees that a triple rhythm is present but finds that the extra sound is louder than either S_1 or S_2. The nursing assessment is that the client's condition has deteriorated even further during the course of the day.

DISCUSSION: Mr. A.'s condition is extremely serious. His level of consciousness is obtunded. The blood-tinged sputum means that tiny bronchiolar capillaries are bursting as a result of CHF. That there is no fever is the only fortunate sign, and it is consistent with the assessment that the origin of the cough is not an infection but rather is cardiac. The alternating pulse detected by the nurse taking the blood pressure confirms severe left ventricular failure and is a very poor prognostic sign. The origin of the S_4 is obscure, but its presence together with the S_3 makes the assessment even more negative. It is especially ominous in that the S_4 had apparently ceased but has now returned. (Of course, the S_4 may have been present in reality but was not heard because the fourth step of cardiovascular assessment was omitted, i.e., contemplation.) The holosystolic murmur is that of mitral regurgitation and is probably functional (i.e., the result of dilatation of the left ventricle, which stretches the valve ring open), but papillary muscle dysfunction, of course, cannot be ruled out. However, the fact that the murmur is soft makes *rupture* of the papillary muscle or septum unlikely. The findings of jugular vein distention, enlargement of the liver, and sacral edema are signs that the failure has extended to the right side of the heart as well. The nurse's assessment that Mr. A.'s condition had worsened during the day is indeed correct. The S_3 and S_4 heard in the morning had blended together to form a summation gallop, which is indicative of severe heart failure.

> Vigorous treatment measures, including the use of vasodilators, are instituted, and by the fifth day Mr. A. is remarkably improved. His respiratory distress is minimal and he is more alert. The alternating pulse can no longer be reproduced. The cough is non-productive. The level of crackles is at the lung bases. The S_4 has disappeared, but the S_3 is still present. A venous pulsation can be seen to throb at the root of the neck. By now, Mr. A.'s physician has become concerned about stagnation of blood and formation of blood clots in the deep venous system after so many days of continuous bed rest and decides to institute anticoagulation measures. An intravenous heparin drip is begun. Some hours later, during an assessment by the nurse, the S_3 is heard faintly and is not audible with every beat. A sound similar to the crunching of boots on snow is heard over the xiphoid process. Careful BP determinations reveal that there is a 6 mm Hg difference in the systolic readings during inspiration and expiration. The jugular pulsation at the root of the neck is still visible. The nurse stops the heparin and telephones the physician.

DISCUSSION: A venous pulsation visible at the root of the neck is a normal finding. There is thus no longer any evidence of right-sided failure in the neck veins. The left-sided failure is dramatically reduced. The crunching-snow sound is a friction rub and signals post-MI pericarditis. Although rubs generally appear before this time in MI, they can occur even later in some cases. The nurse, concerned that the heparin may precipitate a pericardial effusion that could possibly progress to cardiac tamponade, wisely discontinues the anticoagulant pending notification of the physician. Whenever a pericardial effusion develops, the constriction of the heart by the fluid accumulating in the pericardium can engorge the jugular veins and cause a paradoxical pulse. The neck veins are essentially flat, and the 6 mm Hg difference in inspiratory and expiratory systolic pressures indicates normal respiratory variation. These signs therefore do not favor the presence of a serious effusion (more definitive studies, such as CXR, ECG, and echocardiography, would be needed to be certain that none is present).

> By the sixth day neither an S_3 nor a friction rub can be auscultated, and the lungs are clear except for an occasional crackle at the bases. Mr. A. is much more alert, and anticoagulants are resumed. On the seventh day the cardiovascular examination is

entirely normal, and Mr. A. is transferred to the convalescent cardiac unit. After the initial transfer anxiety passes, he begins to enjoy the relative freedom of his new environment. After another three days have gone by, his family notes that his sentences are unusually short and that he is eating very little. He begins to snap at his wife and the nurses over trivial matters. The night nurse records that he had come to the nurses' station at 4:00 A.M. to ask if he could have a cup of decaffeinated coffee.

DISCUSSION: The brevity of speech, anorexia, irritability, and early morning awakening are all clues that the client is becoming depressed.

The nurses on the convalescent unit formulated a plan of care that involved encouraging him to recognize and express his feelings and fears. He eventually revealed that the major concern preying on his mind was the fear of having another heart attack after resuming sexual intercourse. After being reassured that sexual activity could safely be resumed at a certain point in his convalescence, his depression lifted and the remainder of his hospitalization was uneventful. After being discharged from the hospital, Mr. A. joined a final-phase cardiac rehabilitation program, and one year from the date of his MI was healthier than at any other time in his life.

DISCUSSION: Isn't it nice when a story like this has a happy ending?

Bibliography

Abels, L. F.: Mosby's manual of critical care, St. Louis, 1979, The C. V. Mosby Co.

Abrams, J.: Current concepts of the genesis of heart sounds, J.A.M.A. **239:**2782-2791, June 30, 1978.

Andreoli, K. G., Fowkes, G. H., Zipes, D. P., and Wallace, A. G.: Comprehensive cardiac care: a text for nurses, physicians, and other health practitioners, ed. 4, St. Louis, 1979, The C. V. Mosby Co.

Auscultation: are you missing abnormal heart sounds? Patient Care, Nov. 15, 1974.

Barness, L. A.: Manual of pediatric physical diagnosis, ed. 4, Chicago, 1972, Year Book Medical Publishers.

Benchimol, A., and Desser, K. B.: The fourth heart sound in patients without demonstrable heart disease, Am. Heart J. **93:**298-301, March, 1977.

Bouchier, I. A. D., and Morris, J. S.: Clinical skills: a system of clinical examination, Philadelphia, 1976, W. B. Saunders Co.

Carson, P.: Problems in auscultation, Practitioner **220:**370-378, March, 1978.

Champoux, S.: Clinical problems. Part 1. Evaluating patients with acute chest pain, Nurse Pract. **1:**34-37, Jan.-Feb., 1978.

Champoux, S.: Clinical problems. Part 2. Evaluating patients with acute chest pain, Nurse Pract. **1:**30-32, March-April, 1978.

Chung, E. K., editor: Quick reference to cardiovascular diseases, Philadelphia, 1977, J. B. Lippincott Co.

Cochran, P. T.: Bedside aids to auscultation of the heart, J.A.M.A. **239:**54-55, Jan. 2, 1978.

Conn, R. D.: The cardiac examination: an exercise in clinical deduction, Consultant **19:**27-42, Nov., 1979.

Cook, R. L.: Psychosocial responses to myocardial infarction, Heart Lung **8:**130-135, Jan.-Feb., 1979.

Cromwell, R. L., Butterfield, E. C., Brayfield, F. M., and Curry, J. J.: Acute myocardial infarction: reaction and recovery, St. Louis, 1977, The C. V. Mosby Co.

DeGowin, E. L., and DeGowin, R. L.: Bedside diagnostic examination, ed. 3, New York, 1976, Macmillan Publishing Co.

Delp, M. H., and Manning, R. T.: Major's physical diagnosis, ed. 8, Philadelphia, 1975, W. B. Saunders Co.

Dennison, A. J., Jr.: Bedside diagnosis of heart failure, Emerg. Med. **6:**82-85, Feb., 1974.

Eliot, R. S., and Forker, A. D.: Emotional stress and cardiac disease, J.A.M.A. **236:**2325-2326, Nov. 15, 1976.

Fowler, N. O.: Examination of the heart. Part 2. Inspection and palpation of venous and arterial pulses, Dallas, 1972, American Heart Association.

Fowler, N. O.: Cardiac diagnosis and treatment, ed. 2, Hagerstown, Md., 1976, Harper & Row, Publishers.

Friedman, M.: The modification of type A behavior in post-infarction patients, Am. Heart J. **97:**551-560, May, 1979.

Friedman, M. and Rosenman, R. H.: Type A behavior and your heart, New York, 1974, Fawcett Crest Books.

Friedmann, E., et al.: Pet ownership and survival after coronary heart disease, paper presented at the Second Canadian Symposium on Pets and Society, May 30 to June 1, 1979, Vancouver, B.C.

Garrity, T. F., and Marx, M. B.: Critical life events and coronary disease. In Gentry, W. D., and Williams, R. B., Jr.: Psychological aspects of myocardial infarction and coronary care, ed. 2, St. Louis, 1979, The C. V. Mosby Co.

Guyton, A.: Textbook of medical physiology, ed. 5, Philadelphia, 1976, W. B. Saunders Co., chap. 27.

Hackett, T. P., and Cassem, N. H.: Psychological management of the myocardial infarction patient. In Garfield, C. A., editor: Stress and survival: the emotional realities of life-threatening illness, St. Louis, 1979, The C. V. Mosby Co.

Harned, H. S.: Evaluating a child with suspected cardiovascular disease, Consultant **19:**45-47, Dec., 1979.

Harris, A., Sutton, G., and Towers, M., editors: The physiological and clinical aspects of cardiac auscultation, Philadelphia, 1976, J. B. Lippincott Co.

Hartman, R. B.: Pulmonary heart disease: pathophysiology, diagnostic signs, and therapy, Postgrad. Med. **66:**58-71, Sept., 1979.

Hirsch, A. T.: Postmyocardial infarction syndrome, Am. J. Nurs. **79:**1240-1241, July, 1979.

Hurst, J. W., editor-in-chief: The heart, arteries, and veins, ed. 4, New York, 1978, McGraw-Hill Book Co.

Hurst, J. W., and Schlant, R. C.: Examination of the heart. Part 3. Inspection and palpation of the anterior chest, Dallas, 1972, American Heart Association.

Hurst, M. W., Jenkins, C. D., and Rose, R. M.: The relation of psychological stress to onset of medical illness. In Garfield, C. A., editor: Stress and survival: the emotional realities of life-threatening illness, St. Louis, 1979, The C. V. Mosby Co.

Jenkins, C. D.: The coronary-prone personality. In Gentry, W.D., and Williams, R. B., Jr. editors: Psychological aspects of myocardial infarction and coronary care, ed. 2, St. Louis, 1979, The C. V. Mosby Co.

Jeresaty, R. M.: Mitral valve prolapse—click syndrome: etiology, clinical findings, and therapy, Cardiovasc. Med. **3:**597-613, June, 1978.

Leatham, A.: Evaluation of gallop rhythm, Practical Cardiol. **5:**149-160, May, 1979.

Lehmann, J.: Auscultation of heart sounds, Am. J. Nurs. **72:**1242-1246, July, 1972.

Leonard, J. J., and Kroetz, F. W.: Examination of the heart. Part 4. Auscultation, Dallas, 1974, American Heart Association.

Luisada, A. A.: The sounds of the normal heart, St. Louis, 1972, Warren H. Green.

MacBryde, C. M., and Blacklow, R. S.: Signs and symptoms: applied pathologic physiology and clinical interpretation, ed. 5, Philadelphia, 1970, J. B. Lippincott Co.

McIntyre, M. H., editor: Heart disease: new dimensions of nursing care, Garden Grove, Calif., 1974, Trainex Press.

Malasanos, L., Barkausas, V., Moss, M., and Stoltenberg-Allen, K.: Health assessment, St. Louis, 1977, The C. V. Mosby Co.

Moore, S. J.: Pericarditis after acute myocardial infarction: manifestations and nursing implications, Heart Lung **8:**551-558, May-June, 1979.

Moss, A. J.: Heart murmurs: differentiating the innocent from the organic, Consultant **9:**20-23, May-June, 1969.

Neill, C. A., and Haroutunian, L. M.: The ambulatory child with a cardiac murmur, Med. Times **106:**57-60, Nov., 1978.

O'Neal-Humphries, J.: Bedside cardiac diagnosis, Emerg. Med. **10:**25-30, Jan., 1978.

Papenhausen, J. L.: Cardiovascular and respiratory assessment for critical care practitioners. In Current practice in critical care, Vol. I, St. Louis, 1979, The C. V. Mosby Co.

Perloff, J. K.: Concerning the cardiac rhythm called gallop rhythm. In Clinician: congestive heart failure, New York, 1972, Medcom Press.

Petrick, J., and Holmes, T. H.: Life change and onset of illness, Med. Clin. North Am. **61:**825-837, July, 1977.

Ravin, Abe, et al.: Auscultation of the heart, ed. 3, Chicago, 1977, Year Book Medical Publishers.

Riemenschneider, T.: Heart murmurs in infants and children, J. Fam. Pract. **6:**151-155, Jan., 1978.

Sacksteder, S., Gildea, J. H., and Dassy, C.: Common congenital cardiac defects, Am. J. Nurs. **78:**266-271, Feb., 1978.

Segal, B. L., and Likoff, W.: Auscultation of the heart, New York, 1965, Grune & Stratton.

Selzer, A.: Principles of cardiology: an analytical approach, Philadelphia, 1975, W. B. Saunders Co.

Shaver, J. A.: Innocent murmurs, Hosp. Med. **14:**8-28, April, 1978.

Sherman, J. L., and Fields, S. K.: Guide to patient evaluation, ed. 2, Garden City, N.Y., 1974, Medical Examination Publishing Co.

Silverman, M. E.: Examination of the heart. Part 1. The clinical history, Dallas, 1972, American Heart Association.

Silverman, M. E.: The sights and sounds of heart disease, Emerg. Med. **6:**91-98, Feb., 1974.

Slay, C. L.: Myocardial infarction and stress, Nurs. Clin. North Am. **11:**329-338, June, 1976.

Spence, W. F.: Chest pain. In Leitch, C. J., and Tinker, R. V., editors: Primary care, Philadelphia, 1978, F. A. Davis Co.

Stapleton, J. F., and Harvey, W. P.: Heart sounds, murmurs, and precordial movements. In Sodeman, W. A., and Sodeman, W. A., Jr.: Pathologic physiology: mechanisms of disease, ed. 5, Philadelphia, 1974, W. B. Saunders Co.

Stein, P. D., Sabbah, H. N., and Barr, I.: Intensity of heart sounds in the evaluation of patients following myocardial infarction, Chest **75:**679-684, June, 1979.

Stright, P. A., and Soukup, M.: How to hear it right: evaluating and choosing a stethoscope, Am. J. Nurs. **77:**1477, Sept., 1977.

Tavel, M. E.: The systolic murmur—innocent or guilty? Am. J. Cardiol. **39:**757-759, May, 1977.

Turner, R. W. D.: Auscultation of the heart: with notes on observation and palpation, ed. 4, Edinburgh, 1972, Churchill Livingstone.

Walker, H. K., Hall, W. D., and Hurst, J. W., editors: Clincial methods: the history, physical, and laboratory examinations, Woburn, Mass., 1976, Butterworth Publishers.

When your patient has a pacemaker, Patient Care, June 15, 1978.

Williams, R. B., Jr.: Physiological mechanisms underlying the association between psychosocial factors and coronary disease. In Gentry, W. D., and Williams, R. B., Jr.: Psychological aspects of myocardial infarction and coronary care, ed. 2, St. Louis, 1979, The C. V. Mosby Co.

APPENDIX A

Abbreviations used in the text

A_2	Aortic component of second heart sound
AR	Aortic regurgitation
AS	Aortic stenosis
ASD	Atrial septal defect
A-V	Atrioventricular *or* Arteriovenous
BE	Bacterial endocarditis
BP	Blood pressure
CHF	Congestive heart failure
COPD	Chronic obstructive pulmonary disease
CVP	Central venous pressure
CXR	Chest x-ray (film)
DIP	Distal interphalangeal (joint)
DOE	Dyspnea on exertion
DP	Dorsalis pedis (pulse)
ECG	Electrocardiogram
ED	Emergency department
ICS	Intercostal space
IV	Intravenous
JVP	Jugular venous pulse
LBBB	Left bundle branch block
LICS	Left intercostal space
LLSB	Left lower sternal border
LVH	Left ventricular hypertrophy
ⓜ	Murmur
M_1	Mitral component of first heart sound
MAL	Midaxillary line
MCL	Midclavicular line
MI	Myocardial infarction
MR	Mitral regurgitation
MS	Mitral stenosis
MSL	Midsternal line
OS	Opening snap
P_2	Pulmonic component of second heart sound
PDA	Patent ductus arteriosus
PMI	Point of maximum impulse
PND	Paroxysmal nocturnal dyspnea
PS	Pulmonic stenosis
PT	Posterior tibial (pulse)
RBBB	Right bundle branch block
RF	Rheumatic fever
RICS	Right intercostal space
RVH	Right ventricular hypertrophy
S_1	First heart sound
S_2	Second heart sound
S_3	Third heart sound
S_4	Fourth heart sound
STP	Stress/tension/pressure
T_1	Tricuspid component of first heart sound
TF	Tetralogy of Fallot
TR	Tricuspid regurgitation
VSD	Ventricular septal defect
⟶	Think of . . . .

APPENDIX B

Obtaining recordings of heart sounds

A comprehensive set of sound recordings entitled *Heart Sounds and Murmurs* is available free of charge from the National Medical Audiovisual Center (NMAC) of the National Library of Medicine. These recordings were prepared in 1962 by the distinguished cardiologist W. Proctor Harvey, and are made available as a set of nine tapes. The person desiring to obtain them need only send blank audiotape to the NMAC, who will then record the programs on the tapes and return them to the sender.

The heart sounds on these recordings were recorded "live" in actual cardiac cases. Because of this method, some clarity is sacrificed and there is a significant amount of extraneous noise from breathing, muscle sounds, and so forth. However, they do have the advantage of realism in that they reproduce what the auscultator often encounters in the actual clinical situation. In addition, the collection of sounds is exhaustive, and almost all known normal and abnormal heart sounds are cataloged.

Heart Sounds and Murmurs may be obtained by sending blank tapes to the National Medical Audiovisual Center.* Send nine each of the C-60 cassettes or nine each of the 1200 ft reels of $^{1}/_{4}$-inch all-purpose magnetic tape. Allow three weeks for the tapes to be recorded and returned. Send only new, high-quality cassettes or reels.

Recordings made with the cardiac sound simulator present idealized but nevertheless remarkably accurate likenesses of the heart sounds, and using the recordings is an excellent way for beginners to learn the sounds. A highly recommended set of recordings made with such a simulator has been made available by Merck Sharp & Dohme† at the cost of production ($10.00 per set, payable in advance) as a service to health professionals. Each set of cardiac auscultation recordings includes six audio tape cassettes, an explanatory text, and a binder. The program content includes the following:

> *Tape 1:* Side 1—Mitral stenosis
> Side 2—Splitting of sounds and second heart sound

---

*Media Services Section, 1600 Clifton Road, N.E., Atlanta, GA 30333.
†Division of Merck & Co., Inc., West Point, PA 19486, to the attention of Cardiac Auscultation Cassettes, Professional Relations Department.

210

Tape 2:	Side 1—First heart sound and murmurs
	Side 2—Mitral regurgitation
Tape 3:	Side 1—Abnormal and extra heart sounds
	Side 2—Review session no. 1
Tape 4:	Side 1—Aortic valve lesions
	Side 2—Cardiac arrhythmias
Tape 5:	Side 1—Congenital heart disease (Part 1)
	Side 2—Congenital heart disease (Part 2)
Tape 6:	Side 1—Auscultatory phenomena in other diseases
	Side 2—Review session no. 2

Another good resource prepared with the sound simulator is *Heart Sounds and Auscultation: a Heart Sound Tape for Physicians, Nurses, and Medical Students,* by E. Grey Dimond, M.D. Ask for ACCEL supplement tape no. 11, mentioning the title as well. Send $11.00 to the American College of Cardiology Extended Learning (ACCEL).*

---

*Address: 9650 Rockville Pike, Bethesda, MD 20014.

Recording of cardiovascular examination

The following is an example of the recording of a cardiovascular examination of a normal young adult. Note that findings at physical examination that are ordinarily recorded for the listed anatomical regions but that do not pertain to the cardiovascular system have been purposely omitted.

General —alert, oriented, no acute distress
Skin —warm, dry, color good
Pulse —72, regular, amplitude full
BP —120/80 R & Ⓛ arms sitting
Neck —internal JVP 3 cm c̄ client at 45°; carotid pulse contour normal; no bruit or hum
Chest —clear to percussion and auscultation
Heart —precordium quiet; PMI located just medial to MCL in 5-LICS (or not palpable); S₁ single (or finely split); S₂ physiologically split; no S₃, S₄, click, snap, rub, or ⓜ (or, simply, no extra sounds)
Arterial pulses —

	Carotid	Radial	Femoral	DP	PT	(Others used)
Ⓡ	3	3	3	3	3	—
Ⓛ	3	3	3	3	3	—

Abdomen —no bruit or mass; liver percussed at 10 cm in MCL
Extremities —no cyanosis, clubbing, or edema

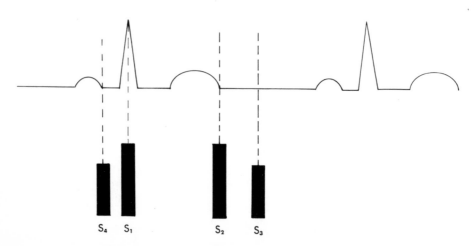

Correlation of heart sounds with electrocardiographic events.

APPENDIX D

Summary sheets

HISTORY

DYSPNEA
1. Shortness of breath
   a. DOE
   b. Positional dyspnea
2. Cardiac cough—nocturnal, precipitated by recumbency, exertion, or side-lying position
3. PND (with wheezing = cardiac asthma)
4. Orthopnea

CHEST PAIN
1. Ischemic: look for pressure quality and radiation
2. "Four E's" of angina: exercise, excitement, eating, exposure to cold
3. P = Provocative-palliative factors: exertion, rest, inspiration or coughing, position, movement, heat, cold, food, drugs
4. Q = Quality: pressure, temperature, sharpness, dullness, tearing
5. R = Region and radiation
6. S = Severity
7. T = Temporal characteristics
8. Cardinal Principle: All chest pain is MI until proved otherwise.
9. Pain of aortic dissection: see summary sheet on aortic aneurysm

PALPITATIONS
1. Life-style?
2. Drug toxicity?

SYNCOPE
1. Effort syncope ⟶ Aortic and subaortic stenosis
2. Stokes-Adams attacks ⟶ Complete heart block
3. Pacemaker syncope ⟶ Pacemaker failure
4. Hypersensitive carotid sinus syndrome

ARTERIAL PULSE

RATE
RHYTHM
FORCE
  0 = Impalpable
  +1 = Feeble
  +2 = Decreased
  +3 = Full
  +4 = Bounding
FORM OF PULSE WAVE
1. Water-hammer pulse—in AR
2. Plateau pulse—in AS
3. Paradoxical pulse—in COPD and constrictive conditions
4. Alternating pulse—in Ⓛ -sided CHF (3 and 4 best detected with BP cuff)
NATURE OF ARTERIAL WALL
1. Unusual firmness (assess in diastole)
2. Tortuosity
3. Bruits (CAUTION: Avoid excessive pressure with diaphragm.)

CLICKS

HIGH-PITCHED SOUNDS
1. Heard best with diaphragm of stethoscope
EJECTION CLICKS
1. Occurrence
   a. In semilunar valve **stenosis**
   b. In great arterial vessel **dilatation**
2. Heard just after S_1 (early systole)
3. Aortic ejection sound—heard best at apex or aortic area
4. Pulmonic ejection sound—heard best at pulmonic area or Erb's point, especially in expiration
NONEJECTION CLICKS
1. Occur in floppy mitral valve syndrome
2. Heard in mid or late systole at mitral area

213

INSPECTION

ORDER
1. Jugular venous pulse
2. Carotid arterial pulse
3. PMI
4. Remainder of precordium

PMI
1. Normal location = 5-LICS at or just medial to MCL
2. Heart rate and rhythm

ABNORMAL PRECORDIAL MOVEMENTS
1. Heave—in LVH
2. Lift—in RVH
3. Pulsations
4. Retractions

PULSATIONS—most common
1. Sternoclavicular area
2. 2-RICS (aortic)
3. 2-LICS (pulmonic)
4. Lower parasternal area
5. Midprecordial area
6. Apex
7. Epigastrium

PALPATION

ALL DISCUSSED UNDER INSPECTION
LVH—THE PMI
1. Shifts leftward and downward
2. Is > 3 cm in diameter
3. Heaves to the Ⓛ
4. Pulsation is sustained

RVH
1. Parasternal lift
2. In cor pulmonale, insert fingertips under Ⓛ costal margin near xiphoid

PALPATION AT BASE
1. Pulsations
2. Thrills
3. Vibrations of heart sounds, especially increased P_2

PALPATION IN OTHER AREAS OF PRECORDIUM AS NECESSARY

PALPATION OF EACH AREA
1. *H*eart sounds
2. *E*nlargement
3. *A*bnormal precordial movements
4. *R*hythm
5. *T*hrills

SIGNS

HEMOPTYSIS ⟶ MS
DEPENDENT EDEMA ⟶ Ⓡ-SIDED CHF

    0 = Absent

    +1 = Trace

    +2 = Moderate; disappears in 10 to 15 seconds

    +3 = Deep; disappears in 1 or 2 minutes

    +4 = Very deep; present after 5 minutes

CYANOSIS
1. Peripheral ⟶ Cold room
2. Central (intraoral) ⟶ Ⓡ -to- Ⓛ shunts

CLUBBING ⟶ CYANOTIC CONGENITAL DEFECTS
1. Floating nail
2. Profile sign—angle < 180° is normal

PERCUSSION

TYPES OF NOTES
1. Resonant—over air-filled lung tissue
2. Dull—over liquid-filled tissue (heart, liver, fluid-permeated lung); extreme is *flat,* heard over solid structures
3. Hyperresonant—over hyperinflated lung tissue (COPD); extreme is *tympanitic,* heard over gastric and intestinal air bubbles and pneumothorax

MURMURS

CAUSES OF TURBULENCE
1. Partial obstruction (stenosis, coarctation, plaques, tumors)
2. Increased flow across normal valve (flow murmur)
3. Backward flow across leaky valve (regurgitant murmur)
4. Flow through septal defect
5. Flow into sharply widened area (aneurysm)

TIMING
1. Systolic (may be innocent)
2. Diastolic (pathological)
3. Continuous (pathological)

INNOCENT MURMUR
CHARACTERISTICS
1. Three S's—short, soft, systolic
2. S_1 and S_2—both normal
3. ECG and CXR—both normal

DESCRIPTION
1. Cycle
2. Configuration
3. Location
4. Intensity (six-grade scale)
   Grade 1—very faint; not heard right away
   Grade 2—soft; heard right away
   Grade 3—moderately loud; no thrill
   Grade 4—loud; thrill present
   Grade 5—very loud; not heard with stethoscope off chest
   Grade 6—loudest; heard with stethoscope off chest
5. Intensity (four-grade scale)
   Grade 1—very soft
   Grade 2—soft
   Grade 3—loud
   Grade 4—very loud
6. Quality—high-pitched, low-pitched, blowing, harsh, rumbling, etc.
7. Radiation
8. Position

INFECTIOUS DISEASES
1. ⓜ + Fever ⟶ BE
2. ⓜ + Fever + Child ⟶ RF

AUSCULTATION

MAJOR LOW-FREQUENCY SOUNDS (HEARD WITH BELL)
1. S_3
2. S_4
3. A-V valve stenosis

ACCESSORY POSITIONS
1. Sitting or standing fully upright—to avoid mislabeling a normal S_2 as a "split S_2 in expiration" in children and young adults
2. Ⓛ lateral decubitus—for detecting S_3, S_4, and ⓜ of MS
3. Seated flexion—for detecting ⓜ of AR and friction rubs

MILD EXERCISE
1. Squeezing fingers
2. Passive raising and lowering of legs
3. Coughing
4. May accentuate S_3, S_4, and ⓜ of MS

CYCLED RESPIRATION
1. Useful technique for detecting sounds that display respiratory variation such as splitting
2. Ⓡ -sided sounds louder with inspiration
3. Ⓛ -sided sounds louder with expiration

INCHING TECHNIQUE
1. Use after S_1 and S_2 have been identified
2. Follow sounds through chest

CARDIAC CYCLE

ORDER FOR LISTENING
1. S_1
2. S_2
3. Systole
4. Diastole

TIMING EVENTS OF CYCLE
1. S_2 louder than S_1 at aortic area
2. Apex beat taps palm as S_1 occurs
3. S_1 coincident with upstroke of carotid pulse

VENOUS PULSE

IF ELEVATED, consider:
1. ℞ -sided CHF
2. Hyperkinetic circulation
3. Fluid overload
4. Constrictive conditions
5. Tricuspid stenosis or regurgitation
6. Obstruction of vena cava

DISTINGUISH CAROTID AND JUGULAR PULSES

Aspect	Carotid	Jugular
Form of pulse wave	Single	Double
Palpation	Felt better with pressure	Impalpable
Inspection	Crisp, discrete	Soft, diffuse
Motion	Up-and-down	In-and-out
Respiratory variation	None	Clearer on expiration
Effect of position	None	Lowering head increases

VENOUS PULSE—cont'd

SPOT ASSESSMENT
1. Elevated if pulsation measures > 1 cm above clavicle with client at 45° angle

ESTIMATING CVP
1. Add 5 cm to JVP

FORM OF PULSE WAVE
1. A wave—caused by atrial contraction; approximately coincides with S_1
2. V wave—occurs at time of ventricular contraction; approximately coincides with S_2
3. If single—usual cause is missing A wave due to atrial fibrillation
4. Large A wave—in resistance to atrial emptying (tricuspid stenosis, pulmonary hypertension) or if atria beat against closed tricuspid valve (junctional tachycardia or 3rd-degree heart block)
5. Large V wave—tricuspid regurgitation

SPLITTING

TIMING
1. 0.00 to 0.02 sec = Single heart sound
2. 0.02 to 0.04 sec = Fine splitting
3. 0.04 to 0.06 sec = (Normally) wide splitting
4. More than 0.07 sec = (Abnormally) wide splitting or extra sound

EVALUATION (doubtful split vs. extra sound)
1. Quality—pitch, loudness, duration
2. Location—splits not heard at sites where extra sounds are heard
3. Timing

GALLOPS

PATTERN OF SOUNDS
1. S_3 gallop: S_1 + S_2 + S_3 ("Kentucky")
2. S_4 gallop: S_4 + S_1 + S_2 ("Tennessee")
3. Quadruple, or cogwheel, gallop: S_4 + S_1 + S_2 + S_3 ("tuh-lubb-dupp-uh")
4. Summation gallop: triple rhythm in which extra sound is combined S_3 and S_4, which is usually louder than S_1 or S_2

AUSCULTATORY AREAS

Name	Location	Major sounds
Aortic	2-RICS next to sternum	A_2 ∴ S_2 usually loudest here Aortic (m)s Aortic ejection click
Pulmonic	2-LICS next to sternum	P_2 ∴ split S_2 heard here Pulmonic (m)s Pulmonic ejection click
Erb's point	3-LICS next to sternum	All sounds of pulmonic area Aortic (m)s Friction rubs
LLSB	4-LICS next to sternum	All sounds of tricuspid area Aortic (m)s Friction rubs OS

AUSCULTATORY AREAS—cont'd

Name	Location	Major sounds
Tricuspid	5-LICS next to sternum	T_1 ∴ split S_1 heard here (R)-sided S_4 (R)-sided S_3 Tricuspid (m)s Friction rubs
Xiphoid Midprecordial area	Around xiphoid Halfway between tricuspid and mitral area in 5-LICS	Friction rubs (L)-sided S_4 in ischemia (R)-sided S_4 (R)-sided S_3 Friction rubs OS

AUSCULTATORY AREAS—cont'd

Name	Location	Major sounds
Mitral	Apex beat	M_1 ∴ S_1 usually loudest here (L)-sided S_3 (L)-sided S_4 Mitral (m)s Aortic (m)s Aortic ejection click OS Nonejection click Friction rubs

FIRST HEART SOUND

LOCATION
1. Loudest near apex
2. Produced by A-V valve closure

SPLITTING
1. Two components: M_1 and T_1
2. M_1 is heard before T_1
3. T_1 is weaker component
4. Split heard best over tricuspid area or LLSB
5. "Wide splitting" more likely to be one of the following:
   a. $S_4 + S_1$ (apex)
   b. S_1 + Ejection click (apex or base)
6. True wide, loud splitting$\longrightarrow$RBBB
7. Loud $S_1 \longrightarrow$ MS ("closing snap")

THIRD HEART SOUND

LOW-FREQUENCY SOUND
1. Heard with bell
2. Ⓛ-sided heard at apex
3. Ⓡ-sided heard to Ⓡ of apex
4. Ⓛ-sided heard best in expiration
5. Ⓡ-sided heard best in inspiration (perhaps also over jugular)
6. Heard in first third of diastole

INCIDENCE
1. One third of persons under 30 years of age normally have S_3
2. If heart condition present or suspected, CHF implied by S_3

ACCENTUATED
1. By Ⓛ lateral decubitus position
2. By hyperkinetic circulation

RHYTHM: "KENTUCKY"

SECOND HEART SOUND

LOCATION
1. Loudest at base
2. Produced by semilunar valve closure

SPLITTING
1. Two components: A_2 and P_2
2. A_2 comes before P_2
3. P_2 is weaker component
4. A_2 is most dominant of all heart sound components
5. Split heard over pulmonic area or Erb's point
6. Split S_2 in expiration is always abnormal (CAUTION: Evaluate with client in upright position before making this statement.)
   a. RBBB
   b. ASD (wide, fixed splitting)
7. Reverse splitting (S_2 split in expiration, single in inspiration)
   a. LBBB
   b. Mechanically-caused LBBB (Ⓡ ventricular pacemaker)
8. **Fix it right** (fixed splitting due to delay in emptying time of Ⓡ ventricle; reverse splitting on "reverse" Ⓛ ventricle)

LOUD $S_2 \longrightarrow$SYSTEMIC HYPERTENSION

FOURTH HEART SOUND

LOW-FREQUENCY SOUND
1. Heard with bell
2. Ⓛ-sided heard at apex
3. Ⓡ-sided heard to Ⓡ of apex
4. Ⓛ-sided heard best in expiration
5. Ⓡ-sided heard best in inspiration
6. Heard late in diastole, just before S_1

INCIDENCE
1. May be normal in late middle-age or older

MAIN PATHOLOGY
1. Ⓛ-sided—systemic hypertension, acute MI or anginal attack
2. Ⓡ-sided—pulmonary hypertension

IMPROVEMENT OF CONDITION
1. Fading of S_4
2. Draws nearer to S_1

RHYTHM: "TENNESSEE"

AORTIC STENOSIS AND SCLEROSIS

SYMPTOMS OF AS
1. Angina
2. Effort syncope
3. DOE

ASSESSMENT IN AS
1. Small, prolonged carotid pulse (plateau pulse)
2. Narrow pulse pressure
3. Aortic ejection click
4. Soft A_2
5. Delayed A_2 (reverse splitting)
6. Signs of LVH
7. Harsh ejection Ⓜ heard best at aortic area or apex, often heard well throughout chest, radiates to carotids

AORTIC SCLEROSIS
1. "50-50" Ⓜ
2. Ⓜ similar to AS except in following characteristics:
   a. Not harsh
   b. Confined to aortic area
   c. Normal carotid pulse
   d. No thrill

AORTIC REGURGITATION

SYMPTOMS OF CHF
ASSESSMENT
1. Bounding, slapping arterial pulses (water-hammer)
2. Wide pulse pressure
3. Signs of LVH
4. Early diastolic, high-pitched, blowing decrescendo Ⓜ ("whiff") best heard at aortic area or LLSB with client in seated flexion position and breath held in full expiration, sometimes accompanied by systolic ejection murmur

MITRAL STENOSIS

SYMPTOMS
1. Dyspnea
2. Hemoptysis

ASSESSMENT
1. "Closing snap" = Loud S_1
2. Opening snap
3. Loud P_2
4. Parasternal lift
5. Rumbling, low-pitched, diastolic Ⓜ
   a. Best heard with bell
   b. Localized to apex
   c. Louder in Ⓛ lateral decubitus position
   d. Sometimes with crescendo accentuation in late diastole (S_1 + S_2 + OS + Ⓜ = "Ffoot-ta-ta-rroo")

MITRAL REGURGITATION

SYMPTOMS
1. Palpitations
2. Symptoms of CHF

ASSESSMENT
1. Soft S_1
2. Signs of LVH
3. S_3
4. Loud, blowing, holosystolic Ⓜ
   a. Best heard at apex
   b. Radiates to Ⓛ axilla

FLOPPY MITRAL VALVE SYNDROME
PROLAPSE OF MITRAL LEAFLET
1. Into left atrium in late systole
2. Gives rise to hallmark sign—nonejection click heard with diaphragm at apex
3. Click may be followed by ⓜ of MR

USUAL PRESCRIPTION
1. Antibiotic prophylaxis against BE

FRICTION RUB
OCCURS IN PERICARDITIS
COMPONENTS
1. Atrial contraction
2. Ventricular contraction (occurs with apex beat)
3. First third of diastole (rapid filling phase)

DIFFERENTIATION
1. Pericardial rub—no variation with respiration
2. Pleural rub—ceases if breath is held

TAMPONADE
1. May be result of anticoagulation agent
2. May produce several signs
   a. Rise in JVP—key sign
   b. Fall in BP
   c. Paradoxical pulse
   d. Tachycardia
   e. Decreased heart sounds
   f. Decreased force of arterial pulses

CONGESTIVE HEART FAILURE
CLIENT WEIGHED DAILY
PATHWAYS OF CONGESTION
1. Ⓛ ventricle ⟶ Pulmonary veins
2. Ⓡ ventricle ⟶ Systemic veins

LEFT-SIDED CHF
1. Reduced forward output
   a. Disorientation (ODD remedy—O_2, Diuretics, Digitalis)
   b. Nocturia
   c. Peripheral cyanosis
   d. Cheyne-Stokes respirations
2. Myocardial decompensation
   a. S_3
3. Enlargement
   a. Signs of LVH
   b. ⓜ of MR
   c. Alternating pulse
4. Increased pressure rearward
   a. Dyspnea
   b. Cardiac cough
   c. Wheezes
   d. Pink-tinged sputum
   e. Crackles
   f. Dullness at lung bases
   g. Central cyanosis

RIGHT-SIDED CHF
1. Reduced forward output
   a. Hepatojugular reflux
2. Myocardial decompensation
   a. Ⓡ-sided S_3
3. Enlargement
   a. Parasternal lift
   b. ⓜ of TR with abnormal systolic pulsations in the venous system (large V waves)
4. Increased pressure rearward
   a. Jugular venous engorgement
   b. Liver enlargement—dullness > 12 cm in MCL
   c. Nausea, indigestion, anorexia
   d. Ascites
   e. Dependent edema

AORTIC ANEURYSM

ASSESSMENT
1. Abnormal pulsations, especially second Ⓛ and Ⓡ ICS, sternoclavicular joints and epigastrium (palpate and auscultate near midline of abdomen for pulsatile mass with bruit.)
2. Loud A_2
3. Aortic ejection click
4. Vascular compression signs
   a. Bilateral or unilateral jugular vein distention
   b. Decreased or delayed arterial pulses
5. Systolic crescendo-decrescendo bruit over site of aneurysm
6. Aortic dissection—pain may have following characteristics
   a. Resemble MI
   b. Have tearing quality
   c. Radiate widely
   d. Migrate outward, inward, or backward

SYSTEMIC HYPERTENSION

ASSESSMENT
1. Loud A_2
2. Signs of LVH
3. S_4
4. Signs of CHF, especially S_3
CURABLE CAUSES
1. Coarctation of the aorta
   a. Pulses of $+3/+4$ in upper half of body; pulses of $+2/+1$ in lower half of body
   b. BP in arms elevated; normal or low BP in legs
   c. Systolic bruit over base of heart or over back or both
2. Renal artery stenosis—systolic bruit in periumbilical region

MYOCARDIAL INFARCTION

ASSESSMENT
1. Decreased heart sounds—acute phase
2. S_4—acute phase
3. Signs of CHF, especially S_3
4. Increased or displaced PMI (may be due to the MI itself, ventricular aneurysm, or LVH)
5. Systolic murmurs
   a. MR—caused by the following:
      (1) Papillary muscle dysfunction (soft)
      (2) Papillary muscle rupture (loud, pansystolic)
      (3) CHF—functional
   b. Septal rupture = VSD (loud, pansystolic with thrill)
6. Friction rub—pericarditis

PULMONARY HYPERTENSION

DEFINITION
Increased pressure in pulmonary artery
CAUSES
1. Chronic cor pulmonale
2. Acute cor pulmonale
3. Ⓛ -to- Ⓡ intracardiac shunts
4. MS
ASSESSMENT
1. Increased P_2 ($P_2 > A_2$)—may be palpable
2. Ⓡ -sided S_4
3. Pulmonic ejection click
4. Systolic ejection ⓜ in pulmonic area
5. Parasternal lift
6. Large A wave in JVP
7. Signs of Ⓡ -sided CHF, especially S_3

CARDIOVASCULAR ASSESSMENT IN CHILDREN

INSPECTION
1. Central cyanosis
2. Clubbing

PALPATION
1. Premature beats and sinus arrythmia (common)
2. PMI
   a. Approximately at age 7 years—assumes adult location
   b. Before age 7 years—may be in 4-LICS up to 1.25 cm (1/2 in) outside MCL
   c. Infancy—4- or 3-LICS up to 1.25 cm (1/2 in) outside MCL
3. Sternal bulging—in RVH

AUSCULTATION
1. S_2—single S_2 suggests congenital cyanotic defect; $P_2 > A_2$ is normal in children; split S_2 in expiration may be normal but should close in upright position
2. S_3—normal in children if isolated finding
3. Innocent ⓜ —short, soft, systolic; S_1 and S_2 normal; CXR and ECG normal; murmur localized (check the back!); BP in arms not higher than in legs
   a. Vibratory ⓜ —at LLSB
   b. Venous hum—continuous bruit in supraclavicular area that decreases if jugular flow is impeded ("30-30" bruit)

CARDIOVASCULAR ASSESSMENT IN CHILDREN—cont'd

AUSCULTATION—cont'd
   c. Pulmonic ejection ⓜ
   d. Carotid bruit—supraclavicular area; systolic ejection bruit

CONGENITAL HEART DISEASE
1. Stenotic defects
   a. Coarctation of the aorta
   b. Pulmonic stenosis
      (1) RVH
      (2) Pulmonic ejection ⓜ —loud, harsh
      (3) P_2 decreased and delayed
   c. Aortic stenosis
2. Ⓛ -to- Ⓡ (A→V) shunts (acyanotic)
   a. VSD—holosystolic ⓜ at LLSB
   b. ASD—possible signs
      (1) Wide, fixed splitting of S_2
      (2) RVH
      (3) No ⓜ
      (4) Pulmonic ejection ⓜ
      (5) Diastolic ⓜ
   c. PDA—continuous, machinery-like ⓜ in infraclavicular area
3. Ⓡ -to- Ⓛ (V→A) shunts (cyanotic)—**single** S_2
   a. Tetralogy of Fallot
      (1) ⓜ of PS may be present
      (2) RVH
   b. Transposition of great vessels—ⓜ if any results from coexisting Ⓛ -to- Ⓡ shunt

APPENDIX E

Answers

MODULE 1

1. Inspiratory
2. Cardiac asthma
3. CHF
4. a. MI
   b. Angina pectoris
5. Pressure
6. a. Exercise
   b. Excitement
   c. Eating
   d. Exposure to cold
7. Pleuritic
8. a. Provocative-palliative factors
   b. Quality
   c. Region (and radiation)
   d. Severity
   e. Temporal characteristics
9. Myocardial infarction
10. Digitalis
11. Aortic
12. Stokes-Adams

MODULE 2

1. Early morning
2. Physical
3. A
4. Overprotect
5. Embellishment; omission

MODULE 3

1. Mitral stenosis
2. Right-sided
3. 3
4. Central
5. Floating nail; profile sign
6. 180

MODULE 4

1. a. Inspection
   b. Palpation
   c. Auscultation
   d. Contemplation

MODULE 5

1. a. Jugular venous pulse
   b. Carotid arterial pulse
   c. Precordium
2. Fifth; midclavicular line
3. Outward; downward
4. a. Heaves
   b. Lifts
   c. Pulsations
   d. Retractions
5. Lift *or* tap
6. Heave
7. Retraction

MODULE 6

1. Left ventricular hypertrophy
2. Left axillary
3. 3
4. Duration
5. Right ventricle
6. Lift
7. Cor pulmonale

MODULE 7

1. Palpation
2. Heart failure
3. a. Dull
   b. Resonant
   c. Hyperresonant
4. Tympanitic
5. a. Pulmonary edema
   b. Pleural effusion
6. Edema
7. 12

MODULE 9

1. Carotid
2. 2
3. A. Probably normal
4. B. Probably abnormal
5. Cessation *or* stoppage; digitalis
6. Aortic stenosis

7. 10; paradoxical
8. Water-hammer
9. Bruit
10. Paradoxical
11. Water-hammer
12. Alternating

MODULE 10

1. Right atrial
2. C. Hypotension
3. A
4. 1
5. A. Propranolol
6. A
7. V
8. Heart failure
9. Emptying
10. Arterial
11. Elliptical

MODULE 11

1. High
2. Bell
3. Hair
4. Firm
5. Atrioventricular *or* A-V
6. Air seal

MODULE 12

1. Blood mass
2. First heart sound
3. S_2
4. Closure
5. Systole
6. Atrioventricular *or* A-V
7. Filling
8. Semilunar

MODULE 13

1. Maximum impulse
2. Secondary aortic
3. Pulmonic
4. Sternum
5. Second; right
6. Mitral
7. Erb's
8. LLSB

MODULE 14

1. c. Systole
   d. Diastole
2. Diastole
3. Upstroke

4. Epigastrium
5. Carotid sinus
6. a. Auscultate at aortic area
   b. Palpate apex beat
   c. Palpate carotid artery
7. Apical

MODULE 15

1. Left; right
2. Inspiration
3. d. Liquid
   b. Bone
   e. Muscle
   a. Fat
   c. Air-filled tissues
4. Fainter
5. Tricuspid

MODULE 16

1. Apex
2. Duller
3. A-V; systole
4. M_1; T_1
5. M_1; mitral *or* apical
6. Tricuspid

MODULE 17

1. Base
2. Sharper
3. All of them
4. Semilunar
5. A_2; P_2
6. Aortic
7. A_2; aortic
8. Pulmonic
9. Base

MODULE 18

1. Fine *or* narrow *or* close
2. *P*
3. 0.02
4. Normally

MODULE 19

1. a. Fourth heart sound
   b. Systolic click
2. C. S_1 does not display consistent respiratory variation.
3. RBBB

MODULE 20

1. a. Aortic *or* arterial
   b. Pulmonary heart

2. Quiet, continuous
3. Right; left
4. Cor pulmonale
5. Expiration; upright
6. Wide, fixed
7. Single
8. RBBB
9. Inspiration
10. Pulmonic
11. Single; split; reverse *or* paradoxical

MODULE 21

1. Filling
2. Bell
3. Apex
4. Right-sided
5. Heart failure
6. A, C
7. First; only
8. Right-sided
9. Left lateral decubitus
10. Hyperkinetic
11. Ventricular
12. Physiological *or* normal
13. Diastole
14. Knock

MODULE 22

1. Atrial
2. S_1
3. Filling
4. Systemic *or* arterial hypertension
5. Low; bell
6. Closer
7. Improving
8. 50
9. Compliance

MODULE 23

1. Kentucky
2. Diastole; S_1
3. Summation
4. S_4
5. Louder

MODULE 24

1. a. Dyspnea
   b. Chest pain
   c. Syncope
   d. Palpitations
2. All chest pain is MI until proved otherwise.
3. CHF

4. a. Provocative-palliative factors
   b. Quality
   c. Region and radiation
   d. Severity
   e. Temporal characteristics
5. B, C
6. Omission; embellishment
7. Right
8. Cold room
9. 5-LICS at or just medial to MCL
10. Palpation
11. a. Left parasternal area
    b. Apical area
12. a. Tympanitic
    b. Flat
    c. Tympanitic
    d. Resonant
    e. Dull
    f. Hyperresonant
13. Duration
14. Carotid
5. a. Alternating pulse
   b. Water-hammer pulse
   c. Paradoxical pulse
   d. Plateau pulse
16. Bruits
17. Right-sided CHF
18. Venous
19. 1
20. a. Venous
    b. Arterial
    c. Venous
    d. Venous
21. a. S_3
    b. S_4
    c. Murmurs of A-V valve stenosis
22. Blood mass
23. a. Diaphragm
    b. Bell
24. Closure
25. a. Apex
    b. 2-ICS to right of sternum
    c. 5-ICS to left of sternum
    d. 2-ICS to left of sternum
26. A-V
27. a. S_1
    b. S_2
    c. Systole
    d. Diastole
28. Aortic
29. First
30. S_3
31. Erb's point

32. Semilunar
33. Lower
34. Right
35. a. Liquid
    b. Air-filled
36. Apex
37. Tricuspid
38. A_2
39. Pulmonic
40. RBBB
41. Inspiration
42. Reverse
43. Right
44. Expiration; upright
45. Cor pulmonale
46. Aortic/arterial
47. Wide, fixed
48. a. S_4
    b. S_3
    c. S_3
    d. S_4
    e. S_4
    f. S_3
49. a. CHF
    b. Systemic hypertension
50. Louder
51. Left lateral decubitus
52. Apex
53. Hyperkinetic
54. Hypertension
55. a. Fading
    b. Approaching S_1
56. CHF

MODULE 25

1. Hold his breath
2. Effusion
3. Tamponade
4. JVP
5. Expiration
6. Two; to-and-fro
7. Ventricular; apex *or* apical
8. Paradoxical

MODULE 26

1. a. Ejection
   b. Nonejection
2. Diaphragm
3. Prolapse
4. a. Pulmonic area *or* Erb's point
   b. Apex (mitral area)
   c. Apex (mitral area)
   d. Tricuspid area *or* LLSB
5. a. Stenosis

   b. Dilatation
6. Mitral valve

MODULE 27

1. Turbulent
2. Thrill
3. B, C, D
4. a. Obstruction
   b. Increased
   c. Backward
   d. Hole
   e. Widened
5. Systolic

MODULE 28

1. Systolic; diastolic
2. Rectangular
3. Diamond
4. Flow
5. Downstream
6. 1/6
7. 5/6

MODULE 29

1. Aortic
2. Left sternal
3. Hyperkinetic
4. Short; soft; systolic
5. Isolated
6. Semilunar
7. Disappeared

MODULE 30

1. Endocarditis
2. Rheumatic fever
3. Vegetations
4. Dental
5. Streptococci
6. a. C
   b. B
   c. A

MODULE 31

1. a. Rheumatic fever
   b. Syphilis
   c. Bacterial endocarditis
2. Stenotic; regurgitant
3. Direction
4. To-and-fro

MODULE 32

1. Runoff
2. Effort syncope
3. Bicuspid

4. B
5. Plateau pulse
6. Paradoxical
7. Sclerosis

MODULE 33

1. Left
2. Ejection *or* flow
3. CHF
4. a. Slow
   b. Fast
   c. Normal
5. D
6. Decrescendo
7. Diastole; stethoscope diaphragm

MODULE 34

1. a. Closing snap
   b. Opening snap
2. Localized
3. S_3
4. S_1
5. Rumbling
6. a. Diaphragm
   b. Diaphragm
   c. Bell
   d. Bell
7. Ffoot-ta-ta-rroo
8. Hyperkinetic
9. Right
10. S_3
11. a. Loud P_2
    b. Lift

MODULE 35

1. Left; functional
2. First
3. Third
4. Axilla
5. Second

MODULE 36

1. Prolapses
2. Nonejection *or* mid-to-late
3. Diaphragm; mitral *or* apical
4. MR
5. Bacterial endocarditis (BE)

MODULE 37

1. a. Output
   b. Decompensation
   c. Enlargement
   d. Rearward
2. Edema

3. Weigh the client daily.
4. a. Pulmonary
   b. Systemic
5. Stretched
6. Regurgitation
7. Wheezes
8. Crackles *or* rales *or* crepitations
9. Breathing
10. Systolic
11. Left-sided failure
12. S_3
13. B, D, E

MODULE 38

1. Right; aortic
2. Arch
3. Arterial; venous
4. Tearing
5. Expansile mass

MODULE 39

1. Second
2. Radiofemoral
3. Fourth; third
4. Aortic
5. a. Low
   b. High
   c. High
   d. Low
6. Fourth
7. A_2
8. Client A (Client B has decreased pulses all over his body and may be in shock.)
9. A
10. D
11. Cerebrovascular
12. Systolic

MODULE 40

1. Artery
2. COPD
3. Cyanosis
4. P_2
5. C, D, E
6. Third

MODULE 41

1. Fourth
2. Third
3. a. Inward
   b. Outward
   c. Outward
   d. Outward
4. B

5. a. Soft
   b. Loud
   c. Soft
   d. Loud
6. B, C, E

MODULE 43

1. Post-MI pericarditis
2. a. Atrial contraction
   b. Ventricular contraction
3. Rise in JVP
4. D
5. A, C, E
6. A
7. Flow
8. a. Very soft
   b. Soft
   c. Loud
   d. Very loud
9. BE
10. RF
11. Friction rub
12. Blood flow; downstream
13. a. C
    b. A
    c. A
    d. B
    e. B
    f. A
    g. B
14. a. Closing snap
    b. Opening snap
15. Rumbling
16. Low; bell
17. CHF
18. S_3
19. B (Since S_2 is normally louder at the aortic area, an S_1 louder than S_2 is an important clue to a closing snap.)
20. C, E
21. Nonejection *or* mid-to-late; click

22. MR
23. Lungs
24. F
25. Asthma
26. a. Right
    b. Left
    c. Right
    d. Left
    e. Left
    f. Right
    g. Left
    h. Left
    i. Right
27. Pulsations
28. Aortic coarctation
29. Systemic hypertension
30. B, E
31. S_3
32. Duration
33. Right ventricle
34. P_2; pulmonic
35. S_4
36. Click; murmur
37. S_3
38. Fourth
39. Aneurysm
40. Papillary muscle dysfunction; CHF
41. Rupture
42. Cyanosis
43. Hold the breath
44. F
45. Cyanotic
46. High; low
47. C, D
48. Lift
49. PDA
50. Holosystolic
51. PS
52. a. MS
    b. MR
    c. AR